I0210247

A Journey Through Male Menopause

(Dream Work)

Poems & Stories
Love words & Hope thoughts
Drawings & Dreams
Active Imagination & Insights to Grow On
&
Reflections on the Wonder of the World

Author: Frank James Michael Costanza
Cover Design: Frank James Michael Costanza
Proofreading: Joan Appleton Costanza

ISBN: 978-1-5323-9727-1
Text Copyright © Frank James Michael Costanza 2018
Tables Copyright © Frank James Michael Costanza 2018
Cover Photo Copyright © Frank James Costanza 1965
Photos Copyright © Frank James Michael Costanza 2018

Dedication

This book is dedicated to the memory of my wonderful parents:

To my mother Mary Elizabeth Carvey Costanza:
without her loving care and guidance throughout my life I probably would not have had the inner Christian strength to survive the events and growth documented here.

To my father Frank Vito Costanza:
without his exemplary model as a Marine, Electronics Engineer and source of guidance throughout my life I probably would not have had the strength of character to become a Marine, the technical drive to study engineering and the persistent desire to teach and provide guidance to future generations.

Preface

An introductory note to this work:

My name is Frank James Michael Costanza. I am an extrovert, a Christian, a Sagittarius, a believer in the Jungian method of dream analysis, a student and teacher of A Course in Miracles, a student of theology and somewhat of an enigma to those whose lives I touch. I believe in the healing power of prayer and inner work, the strength of Christian morals, Christ's teachings on forgiveness and the tenderness of my feminine side. I have written a journal of my dreams, prayers, poetry, writings and self-analysis over the last several years. The result is the book you hold in your hands. After rereading my journey of the past several years, I found myself asking the following question. Is Male Menopause a reality?

After compilation of the following pages of pain, poetry, prose, dreams and growth I have come to the conclusion that male menopause is a reality. I also believe that heartbreaking mid-life crises can amplify that reality and significant growth, both inner and social, can be accomplished with dedication to the process of self-analysis under the guidance of a caring counselor. I was gifted in this life to have come into the acquaintance of Rev. Dr. Robert Stoudt, my counselor, dream consultant and, most of all, dear friend.

My journey through mid-life began with the death of my mother on December 6, 1992. Mom died of a heart attack one week after her and dad's Fiftieth Wedding Anniversary Celebration, a gala event with family friends and renewal of wedding vows. I stood in as dad's best man for the ceremony. It was a memorable party with great fun and laughter. Mom and dad danced the day away with the grace of Fred Astaire and Ginger Rogers. Ten days later mom was laid to rest on my 47th birthday.

Format of this book

This book is divided into four sections:

The Beginning of Pain The deaths of my mother and Uncle Leo, my review of my life's failures and my contemplation of suicide as an escape.

Inner Work My struggle with mid-life (male menopause), dreams and analysis, retreat journals and dream retreats.

Poetry and Prose My poems from the past, poetry from the heart, prosaic writings and lay sermons and temple talks.

Personal Contact with God A visit from Michael the Archangel in my youth. A wonderful experience in the mountains of West Virginia and God's healing of my son Anthony.

The text begins with my mother's eulogy that I wrote and read at her funeral.

Table of Contents

THE BEGINNING OF PAIN

Overview of the Beginning of Pain

MOM's Eulogy was chosen as the start of this chapter because I felt her death and my response to it began the process that I struggled through over the last several years.

From December of 1992 to December of 1993 I struggled with death in many ways. The unexpected death of my mother, the death of my Uncle Leo and the beginnings of the death of my marriage to Jean all caused me to ask what was happening to my life. Why was my world crumbling beyond my control?

The loss of my mother and her burial on my 47th birthday forced me to review my life and to realize my mortality. I had always been invincible in my approach to life up until her death. I lost a wonderful mother, a great counselor and a dear friend. Mom was always there for me, no matter what I asked I could trust her answer.

Uncle Leo, like my father, was the image of a caring and concerned father. An image I hoped I was like in my family. Devotion to my children was what I learned from the men in my family. I began to question why the strong seemed to leave when they still had much to accomplish and share.

Jean's starting to leave our relationship for another in September of 1993 was a crushing blow. I started to have severe bouts of self-doubt and personal criticism that would lunge me into what I referred to in the introduction as male menopause, my passage through mid-life.

I began at this time to fell the inward struggle of life changing me. My belief structure was being challenged on many fronts and I had to perform a sanity check on myself. In my writing to God on the contemplation of suicide, I negated everything positive that ever occurred in my life. This reversal of fact was cleansing in that it allowed me, several months later, to see the inanity of my ramblings.

My work was to be hard but fruitful as I started into counseling

Inner Work

12/09/92 - (My 47th birthday) - MOM's Eulogy

To Dad, my brothers and sisters, our families, relatives and friends:

I would like to speak a brief moment about Mom and God. As our life is a gift from God, so is the very special love and gentleness we receive from our parents their gift to us. Mom was God's gift to her family and friends, she lived her life in the grace and goodness that God wishes all of us to live. She always found a kind word to say, no matter what, she, with Dad, loved us all with the kind of devotion that could never be matched.

Many believe that just before death God flashes us a review of our life for self-examination. I believe that in very special cases such as Mom, God allows a more special preparation as His way of saying thank you for following Him so devoutly. God's gift to Mom was the months of preparation for the 50th Anniversary party last month. He allowed her the unique privilege to review her life at a more relaxed pace with an opportunity to talk with Dad, her children, grandchildren, great-grandchild and friends, in small groups and individually to remember her rich life. The memories that each of us relived these past few months were wonderful. God allowed each of us to share her last moments with laughter, love and great fun. I will always remember Mom with a smile on her face and a gentle "I love you!" on her lips.

Love, Frankie

Inner Work

Notes from the heart at the Catholic Men's Retreat
02/05/93 - God's Blessings in My Life
Jean - Wife, lover companion, friend

Thank you, God, for giving me someone so willing to share life's journey with me. She is my most trusted friend. I can share my deepest feelings, thoughts and fears with her without being brushed aside or turned away. I only wish that I could better express these feelings, somehow these last few years of stress and uncertainty have clouded my thoughts and actions, the feelings I so freely expressed and showed somehow have become hidden from view. I can only pray that Jean can see through the darkness and understand that I am still the same person she met and fell in love with years ago. I do love her and our family so very much. Please God help me to break free from this painful grip the world has on me and let me once again be as outwardly happy as I am inwardly in love.

Jean is love!

Listen with the ear of your heart!

Inner Work

02/05/93 - Things I cannot change (but can learn from)

- The past (my significant failures)
    - leaving IBM
    - PCI failure
    - Hycor failure

- What have I learned from my failures?
    - I do make mistakes (big ones).
    - I <u>can leave</u> them behind if I try.
    - My family's love is my greatest strength.
    - I <u>must</u> look ahead.

- What can I do today to change?
    - Accept the reality of my situation:
        - Wolf Advisory is my job until I find something else so make the best of it.
        - My skills are marketable but marketing takes time.
        - As long as my family is taken care of I should relax.

    - Take control of my life:
        - Adjust my priorities.
        - Admit my shortcomings.
        - Do <u>NOT</u> look for someone else to blame.

    - Enjoy the love freely given by family, friends, etc.
        - Organize my time to allow for the natural flow.
        - Take time to feel, to love, and to be loved.

Inner Work

02/13/93 - A letter to Aunt Rita
on the death of Uncle Leo

Aunt Rita,

At a time like this it is difficult to think happy thoughts and to understand life's burdens, but I know Uncle Leo would want us to enjoy ourselves. I offer you, Sandy, Ricky, Diane, and David my hand to hold on to, my shoulder to lean on or to cry on and my ear to listen to your thoughts. This is a time to reflect on a full, rich life to remember all the good times and put away the bad. I remember fondly Uncle Leo, he always enjoyed life to its fullest. He never brushed any of us aside because he was "TOO BUSY," he always found time for us kids, he was never "TOO BUSY" to share his talents and knowledge with us if we asked him to play in a game, help us build something or show us how. He was always "TOO BUSY" loving and caring, smiling and sharing. I will miss him as I know we all will.

Love, Frankie

Inner Work

Dear God,

Forgive me for my thoughts, words, and the deed I am contemplating. I have listened with my heart for probably the first time in my life to Jean's pain but now I cannot help her with my love because she no longer cares. I wrote here last February about my failures and my pain and how I was going to try harder using Jean's love as my strength to help me. I failed again. I have been reviewing my life these last few days and the outlook for the future. My life has been a litany of failures that I called triumphs. I was a less than average student, but I always found a way to blame the teachers or the fact that I never stayed in one place long enough to establish myself. I told the world this gave me great insight WRONG!! It just gave my ego a boost. I was a Marine and have used that as some emblem of great strength WRONG AGAIN! I was a less than average Marine, I was busted twice for stupidity. I never finished the career I thought I started. I saw lots of death. I saw a friend blow his brains out because of failure to qualify on the rifle range and thought at the time what a waste, but now I understand why he did what he HAD to do. His failure was his last failure he had to face. Another friend did the same when he didn't make a promotion he deserved. I thought him stupid because I didn't make the grade several times but kept going on, but now I see I was failing to understand his need to escape failure. My cousin Joe killed himself over the loss of love of his wife and I did not understand it but I do now I can feel his need to release himself from the frustrations of constant failure. I realized this morning that instead of a life of successes mine has been one of continued failures. I was always too caught up in what I understood as success to see or admit my abject failure. I could not be wrong. WRONG, WRONG, WRONG!!! I usually was wrong but not man enough to admit it. Now that I see the truth no one else wants to hear me. I have an appointment to talk to a counselor about my feelings, but I do not know if I will be around to make it. Please forgive me for planning my death but you and I have had this conversation many times before only there was someone here to help me through. I look back on our eighteen years and see more clearly now my failures. I never fully understood why when I was in the house there was chaos, but it was always true. This morning I stayed home from work and as usual my presence upset the routine and caused trouble. This has been true for the last eighteen years. Jean always managed to get

6

the children ready better without me. When I come home from work an otherwise peaceful household becomes chaos. I am a failure as a parent. I always considered myself a great father, spouse, son, brother WRONG!!!! I am the ultimate joke upon which laughter does not fall. My list of failures I wrote during the retreat was only the tip of the iceberg. As I see more clearly now my failings, I look to you for help. Jean no longer can or wants or cares to help and I don't blame her. She is right I do try to explain everything to make it better but if I can't explain it to myself to make it better, I fail again. I wish mom was here to help me she always knew what to say or how to make me feel better. I realize now why Uncle Leo's death hurt so much. He was the type of father everyone dreams of, always doing things with his kids always with time for everyone. I am too much like my dad. He was always busy, constantly on trips, taking night courses to better his lot in life but to what avail, to have us kids take advantage of all that he had and not give much in return. After mom's death we did not understand dad's need to move on and we tried to find fault with his relationship with Gloria. I guess we felt we knew it all WRONG. As I look at the similarities in us, I know why Jean felt anger at me when dad started dating she saw dad in me and didn't like it because I was going to have a ball after she died. I think I can eliminate that feeling for her by going first. and since her love for me does not exist my leaving will not hurt. Children somehow know their parents will die someday but don't expect their friends, sisters, lovers, etc to die, so my death is an inevitable occurrence in their life. My ego always told me I was needed in their lives WRONG!!! Every time I tried to help in their lives I was rejected and told to not interfere. Why didn't I understand this until now? Jean told me often to leave them alone and let then struggle and make it on their own, but I would not listen. God, I miss Jean's love. I hurt so bad, worse than I ever did before maybe that's why my thoughts of suicide never fully matured. They needed time to nurture, loss and pain are great fertilizers. I can not continue to lie to myself I need help but there's no one there, I need love, but I killed it, I need, I need, I need but I let it all slip through my grasp. I can't write anymore I even fail to complete my thoughts. I cannot think of the best way to fulfill my task at hand, so I will probably fail at that and not only have to face more pain and emptiness but will have lost my soul in the process. Please help me, please, please, please.

Inner Work

11/10/93 - Another morning of failure

Another morning of failure. I tell Jean I am going to stop my daily stops at the Club because I saw it as one of the problems in our relationship and I am told I am WRONG although in her explanation of the causes of our problems the other day she said I was never there. The contradictions are very confusing to me. I am still here because I have things I must compete before I leave. When I try to make changes to better our way of relating to each other I constantly hear "I FEEL NOTHING!" On the way to work I screamed out in anger at the futility of all my efforts. I have noticed the greatest change in Jean since the continued presence of her cousin Jack. I like Jack, I think he has a good heart, <u>BUT</u> I also feel he is filling the void of his failed marriage and his son being away by using my wife and son as surrogates. Can't he see that this is destroying our family. If he cares for my wife and family, why can't he be a force that is positive rather than a means of escape for Jean? Why can't he and Jean see that the greatest force creating the gap between Jean and I at this time is his providing not an avenue for healing and open discussion that could help (and I desperately need help) us rather than a resounding:

Yeah Jean, Frank is a losing proposition for you. We can have fun, Tony and I have fun but we DON'T NEED FRANK AROUND BECAUSE HE'S NOT FUN!!!

I have got to finish my tasks, I must have a nice weekend with the girls, I must try Monday's session with Dave, I must have my operation, so I will be a pretty corpse. I don't want to look bad when I leave. I must say goodbye to the family by being there at Thanksgiving because I feel that it is the last time, we will really all be together as a family. I must visit mom's grave and let her know I'll see her soon. I am not sure about December I am not sure if my birthday will be something to celebrate or to mourn. I cannot see as far as Christmas. I am not sure it is in my future as each day goes by with another affirmation of Jean's lack of love for me, I die a little more. I don't know when I will cease to function, but I know it is not far in the future. I know that Jean and the kids will be well off. They will have no house payments, no major bills and Jack will be able to fill my void as I have been a void for so long already. I cannot say anything to Jean to let her see my love for her. Everything I say gets thrown back at me "Don't call me that your dad called your mom that." My dad constantly told my mom she was beautiful as I have told Jean. Only now I am not allowed to say those things because dad said them. I have racked my brain to find a phrase to say that my father never used to honor my mom but there aren't many. I refer to Jean as my bride, dad did the same to mom, so I am WRONG. I call Jean pretty or beautiful or gorgeous or lady and I am WRONG because dad said it too. Jean constantly refers to the "Cats in the Cradle" and it is true I have grown up like my dad, but until mom's death showing love to Jean as often and as deeply as dad did to mom was OK. Now it is WRONG. I cannot win, if I try one thing I "shouldn't change my life." But life isn't perfect we all compromise to work and live together. We are not islands, we must touch, share, bend, make changes, care. I am exhausted. I love Jean, I love Jean, I love Jean.

INNER WORK

Explanation of Inner Work

Inner Work is a Jungian approach to using dreams and the imagination for a journey of inner transformation. Under the tutelage of Dr. Robert (Bob) Stoudt, Pastor of Penbrook United Church of Christ, Harrisburg, Pennsylvania, I began my Inner Work of transformation as I struggled with a year of personal loss. The passing of my mother and her subsequent burial on my 47th birthday along with my wife's announcement nine months later of no longer wishing to be married caused me to start questioning my world and its validity. Bob introduced me to Jungian analysis through his "Dream Retreats" at Wernersville Jesuit Retreat Center. His guidance allowed me to take a much deeper look at myself, my relationships and my connection with my God. His format of searching for healing dreams using the Asclepian method of dream analysis at silent "Dream Retreats" was the cauldron that started my central transformative experience.

The Yearly Dreamwork Journals in the following sections are transcriptions of:

- Dreams
- Analysis of said dreams
- Active Imagination
- Personal observations
- Contemplative retreats
- Counseling sessions with analysis
- Conversations with friends and acquaintances
- Introspective analysis of myself and my reactions to life's challenges
- Honest, personal and sometimes painful self-realizations

Inner Work

1993 DREAMWORK PROSE and POETRY
Overview of 1993

The year 1993 was the beginning of my transition through what I call male menopause.

In the "Beginnings of Pain" chapter you read how I started the year with the Catholic men's retreat to gather my thoughts after my mother's death in December of 1992 and to review where I was in life.

In early September my life started to change due to external forces, specifically my wife's announcement that she no longer wished to be married. I tried to rationalize her actions as her going through menopause and began denying my own changes.

This shift led to my contemplation of suicide and my beginning of counseling sessions with Reverend Doctor Robert Stoudt. My first reaction to the changes around and within me was to write a letter to God asking forgiveness for my plans of suicide and taking all my high points of my life and career and negating them all mentally. This process allowed me to reach a depth of personal despair that fostered the inner growth that was to begin.

My continual search for inner peace coupled with Bob Stoudt's recommendation that I begin journaling my dreams gave birth to the document you hold in your hand and set the stage for my intense three-year journey through male menopause. The guidance I received from Bob Stoudt kept me focused and, more than likely, alive throughout my ordeal.

Books recommended by Bob whetted my appetite for information on the inner self and I became a voracious reader. The decision to follow a Jungian method of dream work was fostered by the many books I read written by Robert A. Johnson. His writings were to become the foundation for my inner work and my pathway through mid-life.

12/02/93 - Long Session with Bob Stoudt

I had a long session with Bob Stoudt yesterday. He is very easy to talk with and he hears me. I also talked a lot with Jean today about my conversation with Bob yesterday and her talk today, she is so hard, her mind has really closed me out. I am even more confused now than ever before. I told Bob my perception of the last few years was wrong that now I see better what I did to cause Jean's loss of love for me. I am afraid of sleep now as I do not want to dream. After Viet Nam my

11

dreams kept me without rest. I don't want those dreams to return but as I told Bob my years of "survival" lately are very similar to how I got through the war. I immersed myself in my labors to avoid the horrors of war and then I did the same to avoid the reality of economic disaster impending. The war I could not stop nor the economic disaster. I am either gifted or cursed by God with a strong ability to sense the near future, but no one listens to me. In Viet Nam the military structure of command did not allow me to tell those in control what I saw coming so my friends and I discussed things, wrote letters, burnt those letters and watched in horror as the insanity continued. In my professional career I was better heard. I was considered one of the best technically in IBM. Good enough to be allowed to leave the lab into marketing to help them address the new reality of networks and PCS. Yet the structure of the IBM marketing division was the same as the military. I was in another war, once again trying to survive yet this time NO ONE listened. I knew the direction the market was turning from my project work in the labs. I tried to warn marketing, but no one cared, I was "Plant Life," not a real marketing person. I went to a stockholder meeting in the spring of 1987 and tried to warn the top management, I talked to John Opel and Cap Kastrani for some time and they seemed to listen. A one-time response from Armonk really put me in jeopardy. I was shifted to the Customer Center by management where I could "Demo" equipment but not affect the marketing cycle. Why was I unheard? I saw the handwriting on the wall, but new management tried to build a case to have me fired I had to get out while I still had some integrity. I went up the chain of command and requested an early retirement option and got it from Sal Faso. I warned him and others of the impending destruction IBM was facing if they did not change now. Why did they not listen to me? So many people out of work, losing security and facing financial ruin. I am learning that I do not communicate as well as I thought or I might have helped prevent IBM's demise or at least soften the blow. A friend of mine quit IBM at the same time as I did. I was looking for employment opportunities at the same time he was starting a business. He knew my technical capabilities and insight and a deal was struck. He and I went out to "Network the Nineties." He was a marketer with the future in his hand. We immersed ourselves in an uphill battle against the status quo. Multiple tragedies in his wife's family caused him to cease to be capable of functioning so I found a way to buy him out and take over control. At last I could control my destiny or, so I thought. I was back at war only this time I had no safety net, no fallback position, it was do or die, succeed or face disaster. I did well for a year then I saw an opportunity to do a joint project with IBM, my old support base. I did not remember how it had been when I was there in marketing because this time I held some of the cards only IBM held the Aces and their usual slow response to a golden opportunity turned a potential for great success into a crushing defeat for me. Once more I was in the middle of a battlefield against the odds. Deeper and deeper I went into myself to try to find a solution that was beyond my grasp. I am now really in the war, me trying to survive, no friends in this war, I was alone in my struggle. I crawled deeper into my bunker and tried to prevent the inevitable only this time there were no letters home to burn, no way out. I tried everything to make it work and failed. I caused great suffering instead of preventing it and now I must pay. I found a buyer for the business, we merged, and his arrogance did not allow him to listen to me either and we also failed, now I was broke, in debt and on unemployment. Eight months of searching everywhere produced only one real job, Wolf Advisory, a company who said the needed my talents and vision. I was to become a worker bee in a very busy hive only to be once again unheard. Deeper I crawled into myself, I became a true workaholic, totally avoiding the confrontations of family life. Desert Storm came and went, and I had to visit "The Wall." I had to face my nightmares "Did Larry Kalama die in my arms" or was it something else that happened in the jungle of Viet Nam. Much to my relief Larry's name was not there but now I face a new quandary, "What really happened back there?" I sluff off the question and bury myself deeper in my struggle for survival. I am now a fighting machine, the war rages on around me and I must survive. Recent lost battles emerge as court battles, Corporate Bankruptcy, Personal Bankruptcy, all these trials I must face alone as Jean refuses to go with me for the first time in my life I must really stand alone in a struggle for survival and I am lonely. I have created a void into which I jumped and now cannot get out of. I ask for help, but Jean is beyond my reach and I must fight alone, no reinforcements, no armor, just me, just like the time in the jungle, my helicopter above and me down below shooting at anything that moved. My escape route closed by my own personal barrage only in the war I ran out of ammo and was pulled home to safety by my friends. Now I have no friends and the ammo is my closed mind and open mouth. It is time for a wake-up call and Jean gives me one only it's not what I want to hear. I want mom's reassurance that everything will be OK only mom is dead and Jean says wake up Frank my love for you is dead. I have killed what I was trying to rescue. I destroyed my best friend, I killed a great partnership. I destroyed Jean's love. I will burn in Hell for my sin, I killed a precious gift from God. Who else did I destroy? What happened in the jungle? Did I kill my own friends? God help me to remember, help me to make amends. Why did the pilot stay up there and leave me alone? I don't remember I was only told about what they saw from above, I was shooting into the jungle at something or someone. It was unsafe for them to land. What did I do that was so terrible that my mind refuses to let remember? Did I really hold someone in my arms as they died?

Was it all a dream or a horror too painful to face? I don't know, I need help, I need Jean's love and strength. I am a child alone in a war for survival. God help me! I hurt deep into my soul. I need a strong hand to hold and to guide me, but my ego killed the care felt by Jean. I cannot write any more, I am exhausted, I need release from this. I am the cause and the effect, I am alone.

12/06/93 - The Cats in the Basement

Jean has always reminded me of the song "The Cats in The Cradle" to try to wake me up to the world around me. I started to listen this spring and worked hard to change both myself and the conditions in which I was entrapped. My ultimate success resulted in further closing Jean's soul. I once again engulfed myself in a task I thought necessary and charged the barricade with a full head of steam but forgot to let those around me know of the impending struggle. I heard the cries of Jean and they fueled my passion to succeed with the task at hand. I misunderstood what Jean was saying. I failed to see that the harder I fought to change my work situation the less I gave to her and the kids. I look back now with regret and ask for forgiveness, but no one hears me. I can paint two pictures to illustrate what I feel. The first one is the scene of Renee and I returning from confirmation retreat. We were so high on God's love and our shared experience that Jean and the others were wondering what we had shared that was so uplifting. We shared our weekend with Jean and the others and they felt our enthusiasm to some degree but could not fully feel what we had felt because you "had to be there" to get the full impact. Recently Jean went on a "Cousins Tour" to Ocean City. She and Jack came back higher than a kite while Sara, Char and Mary Lou looked like Hurricane Agnes rolled over them. I asked Jean how the weekend was and all I was told was "Jack and I had a great time, but the others were angry." I heard no more about the fun she and Jack shared only the bad times the others had. Jean did not want to share her happy moments with me as Renee and I had with her and I felt hurt. The following weeks were filled with Jean and Jack having fun, going out, he came over and they walked and talked together, and I was not allowed in to share their happiness. I was being slowly removed from any ability to share Jean's happiness and I retreated into myself and became less and less a burden to Jean's life. I should have stood up and said, "Wait I want to enjoy this high too, but I kept quiet until Jean finally crushed me with her announcement that she did not feel love for me anymore. I feel like the cats in the basement. Our cats had the run of the house in New York, they played with the dog, the kids and us and just had fun. We moved here and rather than a source of love and happiness they became a threat to the material possessions we surrounded ourselves with, so we made the basement their domain. Our dogs, Moxie and Lady, were given reign over the living area but the cats were shut out. They scratch at the door for attention and Jean tells one of the children to go down with them and play. The cats hear us love and cajole with Moxie and Lady, but they are left alone. I am scratching at the door of Jean's heart. Jack and Sara are Moxie and Lady. Their needs and feelings are more important than mine. The more I scratch the more I am ignored. I had a real bad night the other day and Jean held me and talked to me and cared for me as she hadn't done for a long time. I went to Bob to talk about my pain. I now realize that it is not the Viet Nam war that is tearing me up but the emotional war I am fighting now. There is more at stake now than there was then, so I feel the pain more acutely. Mom died a year ago today, I wept last night, Jean held me close to comfort me. God she can make me feel so good, so safe, so loved. Even now when she says that there is no more for me, when I am in deep pain about things other than us she can hug me and make me feel loved and cared for. I miss her so much. We made an agreement the other day. We would try staying in the same house, but we would give each other space whenever the other needed it. It is hard not to touch, to hug, to inquire when someone you love seems to be elsewhere but this we must do to allow each other to grow. I pray for God to strengthen me in this. I do not like being the cats in the basement I want the door opened and the ability to feel the warmth once again. I am willing to learn, to try, to let go and let God, to love, to share and to care.

Inner Work

12/11/93 - My Enlightenment Concerning Myself

I slept last night, soundly for the first time I can remember. The alarm woke me from my dreams and I just wanted to let the pillow engulf me and take me back to rest. My conversation with Jean after Renee's call caused many things to gel in my mind and the sleep finally came to me. My struggle has been being fought forever it seems. I was right the other day when I wrote I am the cause and the effect. My decision of 31 years ago was to haunt me forever. A brave, bold youth with a heart full of compassion entered the military to test his convictions. I am afraid the choice has been my ultimate demise. My 17-year-old psyche was not really emotionally ready for the next four years of gut-wrenching reality. I was a child of love and feeling who thrust himself into a cold and heartless environment, but I survived or did I? Four years of soulless life left a deep scar that never healed. It is now time to heal. I feel great today, the best I have felt in years. I reread my earlier writings and things started clearing up. The years of helping Jean with her group sessions were great escapes from what was inside me. I could help her, hold her, care for her but what about me. Why didn't I help myself rather than bury more pain and resentment inside? I want release from my mental process, but Jean and Bob say that those processes help the ultimate outcome. Birth is painful, I watched both of my sons and my grandchildren inflict deep searing pain on my wife and daughter during labor then saw the total relief and happiness come over them as their latest child was put into their arms. I am feeling the pains of my inner labor now and hope the relief comes soon. I do not like pain. I inflicted great pain on a loving child 31 years ago and now I must give that child back his life. Yesterday was very painful but full of growth. The realization that Bob Anderson was having nightmares about Viet Nam also prodded something in my mind. Then relating Renee and Lee Ann's attitudes towards Jean to Jean really kicked in the old gray matter. I did not try to do my usual logical sequence to analyze the hell out of my feelings rather I let my dreams work out. I don't really remember what I dreamt last night only that I awoke refreshed mentally and emotionally drained. A great weight had been lifted off my chest and I feel I can breathe without thinking about it once again. I must ask Bob this week to help me find out what happened to me. It is a beautiful day today. Jean and I shared the beauty of the moon and clouds in the early dawn and it felt good.

Inner Work

12/12/93 - Young Boy in Church (dream)

Awakened by a dream. I am a young boy 7 - 10 years old. I am being called to step forward. I am in a room full of people either an auditorium or a church. As I walk from the rear of the seats toward the front I notice that I am naked, and the people are all people I know today staring at me and I wake up. I think the people were in pews or benches not individual chairs. I could not really see the whole of the room only myself naked in the aisle walking with people I know looking on. No one seems shocked at my nudity.

12/13/93 - Football Coach (dream)

Awakened again by the alarm from a dream. I am in a football game where we keep playing the same play over and over. the coach's voice is Jean's. I finally call time out and tell the players to just run the play the way the coach said to, no short cuts, no changes, just follow the plan. We run the play exactly as directed, the pass is complete, and the receiver is running toward the goal. The alarm wakes me before I know if we were successful.

12/13/93 - Personal Review of Last Two Days

These last two days were very productive and uplifting. Jean and I talked Saturday and Sunday and I started to realize what was happening within me. Jean is very helpful and supportive of my process although I feel I must not use her strength so much. I may be causing her undue stress and confusion. She needs her own space and time to refresh herself. We learned a lot about each other these last two days. Last night I thanked Jean for her attentive ear and told her it was nice to meet her. She is really a beautiful person inside and out. I pray that we can come to some sort of reconciliation of our differences to allow us to restart fresh together. I must deal with all that I have discovered these past two days and try to learn who I really am. I have asked both our daughters to lay off their mother as I have to resolve my conflicts with myself before I can really deal with the present conflict with Jean. God do I hate confrontation, it is the one task I loathe and avoid at all cost.

17

1994 DREAMWORK PROSE and POETRY

Overview of 1994

The year 1994 began with dealing with the anger I felt as a result of my marriage of 18 years crumbling. My internal and external admission of a struggle with the male ego provided Psyche a platform on which to launch my intense dream sequences.

The 40 or more dreams and active imagination recordings throughout 1994 showed my struggle and growth. I had many ups and downs but overall, I continued to grow in spirituality and self-respect. I was greatly inspired by M. Scott Peck's book "The Road Less Traveled."

My "Journey Inward Dream" in March was presented to me during a dream by Seth, third son of Adam and Eve, and inspired the two poems, "The Journey Inward" and "The Dark Side of the Isle" included in the poetry section of this book.

In an effort to come to grips with my internal changes and the intensity of the dreams I was having, I went on a directed personal retreat to The Jesuit Spirituality Center in Wernersville, PA. This silent retreat into myself and away from my external turmoil provided me with a stronger drive and desire to push on through my process. The Novitiate was a very therapeutic environment with my many emotional levels becoming more invigorated. I found an internal peace there that enhanced my work and helped prepare me for the rest of the year. I also felt a reaffirmation of an inner call for spiritual work that I had denied for years. My life and outlook were to change that spring never to be the same again. I thank my personal director, Father Jack Barron, for his support and guidance while on retreat. He continues to be a friend and source of strength in my life. Wernersville was to become my place of sanctuary and inner growth, a place to which I would return many times when in need of peace.

I began to read "A Course In Miracles" by the foundation of Inner Peace and my life found new meaning. I began a regimen of study that would change my outlook on life and enhance my Christian belief in unconditional forgiveness. I am now a student/teacher of the course.

The next two months were to be full of dreams of growth and introspection and my realization that my marriage was finished. I thank Jean, Jack and Bob Stoudt for their parts in my process, without whom I would not have been stretched so far nor given cause to grow so much. Through pain many blessings were nurtured.

18

Inner Work

The summer of 1994 brought Bob Stoudt's first "Dream Retreat", an exercise in the Asklepian method of incubating a "healing dream." I began to hone my ability to journal my dreams and develop an ability to awaken with more detail than before. This weekend was to begin a shift in my inner work and my dreams. My dreams began to direct me more toward where I was going to rather than where I had been. I felt the transition from a deep feeling of inner guilt and hopelessness to one of growth and fulfillment. I was beginning to grow, and it felt good. The sense of God's presence in my life was intensifying.

My continued study of "The Course in Miracles" and the application of Holy Spirit's teachings to my daily life gave me new hope and strength to go on with my life.

The fall of 1994 I would write "Musings on Death", a hopeful perspective on handling the death of a loved one. I dedicated it in memory of my mother and presented it to a young woman whose grandmother recently died. It was to become a beginning of my helping people through the grief process.

I exited 1994 whole and full of life, ready to take on the world. I could not contain my exuberance within, my love of life became infectious to those around me.

Inner Work

01/08/94 - Enraged, can't sleep

Enraged, can't sleep, full of anger, I hate Jack for giving Jean that damn stuffed animal. It is a permanent reminder of her affair with Jack and a constant barrier between us at night. She does not sleep without it. I touched her back tonight and she recoiled and pushed my hand away. I was told to turn over, so I would not snore the she rolled over and crammed that damn animal into my back as she went to sleep. I want so desperately to do all that was talked about in our session with Bob Friday. Anthony asked Jean today if we could just forget our troubles and start going to church again at our own church as a family. She told me she had a lot of thinking to do concerning that then she went out with Jack and Sara for the day and returned after eleven. I try so hard to contain my emotions, but I love Jean so much that when she is not here, I have such searing loneliness that I cannot function. I want our relationship back, I want her love. I am tired of being rejected, cheated on, made a fool of, and just plain being hurt. Why can't I accept the fact that Jean does not love me, does not want me, and only needs me as a source of basic needs of survival which of course she reminds me Jack or Sara would provide if need be. I am in a horrible losing proposition, if I demand a decision, I am forcing her to make a possible wrong choice although she has never wavered over the last five months in her denial of love for me. I am still a man full of love for Jean and a great desire to have my sexual needs fulfilled. I do not know how long I am supposed to allow myself to be used like this. I am afraid my rage may blow out some day soon and then I will have hell to pay. God please help me!!!

Inner Work

01/10/94 - Advanced Calc (dream)

In college going to Advanced Calc class. I didn't attend often. Student said Dr. Terry was late, but I shouldn't be there because I missed so many sessions. I looked at the complex problem on his sheet and told him the answer. Dr. Terry appeared (history teacher), I left room because he did not belong. Ran to men's room somebody followed me and gave me a long stick. Anthony appeared asking me to do something, I said OK and started to follow. Went back for the stick it was perfect for a walking stick. I was on top of a hill behind a house talking with friends and looked down at the house below, Jean came out to beckon me to come home. I started down the hill towards her and she disappeared. I was looking over some trees planted by a friend next to a large wall (stepped) the other side of the wall was deep. Anthony and I were at the bottom painting something bright yellow. A construction crew came to fill in the space between the wall and the other side. We watched as they pushed mounds of dirt into the hole. The dirt started to cover the yellow object and Anthony began to cry. I screamed at the bulldozer operator to stop, then demanded the crew remove the dirt that was covering our work. The workers began carefully shoveling away the dirt and it seemed like it would take an eternity to complete the task as I watched them work with my walking stick in one hand and my arms around Anthony I work up.

01/10/94 12:30 PM - Lunch time short conversation

Lunch time short conversation with Jean. She still feels she did absolutely nothing wrong in respect to our relationship, everything just happened last year therefore everything after her feeling of no love was OK. Even though I was never told anything until after the fact. How do I deal with this? Extrovert versus introvert communication. Hope or hopeless.

01/10/94 04:45 PM - Another enlightenment occurs

Another enlightenment occurs. I realize that Jean's internal peace is a great comfort to her. Although I am still struggling with my male ego I am learning a lot. From Jean's point of view having her "affair" with Jack was not wrong because she feels nothing for our relationship. From my point of view, it is wrong since we are still married and have not formally called it quits. One can rationalize either position as correct depending on their individual perspective. In today's legal system my view would be taken in the world of pure individualism both views are correct, and a solution would be hard to come by. A compromise would have to be made but by whom and which one must swallow his or her pride to bring balance to the situation? I feel much more at ease now and I look forward to my session with Bob tomorrow. I also am anxious for Jean to set the time and date for our next session with Bob as she says she will set it when she is ready to open up to me more on what emotional needs are left unmet. This next session could be the key to either reconciliation or divorce, but I know now that we are coming closer to that critical point in which we come to that fork in the road.

01/11/94 - My Fire Dream

Awakened by a dream. We are at a sports event in a stadium in a valley surrounded by a forest. During the event we (Jean, Mike, Tony and I) notice a fire off in the distance but think nothing of it. As time goes on we notice the fire is getting larger and that it is a forest fire that will eventually engulf the whole stadium area. Mike and I leave Jean and Tony at a safe area near the access road to the parking lot and go to get the car. As we walk to the car the fire has started to surround the whole area. Everyone is trying to get to their cars now. Mike and I get to the car and drive down to pick up Jean and Tony. We are all in the car safe but all around us is mayhem and the fire is now raging beside the road as we drive away and I wake up as we are looking from our car on a ridge overlooking the stadium and watch the roaring inferno.

01/14/94 - A Tennis Lesson (dream)

I am sitting waiting for a tennis lesson. I come in as Jimmy Conners to teach myself how. When I speak, I sound like Jimmy, but I know it is me teaching myself. I learn rapidly then thank myself (Jimmy) in my own voice. I leave to go to work from there, am going up a steep mountain. There is a long line in front of me as traffic is slowed down for construction. I arrive at work where I am being put through orientation on the top floor of a new building, unfortunately the elevators are being worked on, so I must take the stairs up to the eleventh floor. They group us in threes to fill out forms, mine are already done and I am put in charge of helping the others fill theirs out then all of a sudden, I am in a beautiful field with friends playing cards. The guy dealing keeps misdealing and dropping cards, we never get a hand started but I am very relaxed and enjoying myself. I wake up.
When traveling before the traffic jam. I approached the area and saw a policeman on the left (radar I thought) and I noticed I was not speeding but the officer was waving people to slow down and get in the right lane. I stayed in the left and passed everyone and no one seemed

22

angry about my passing to the front.

Also, the person passing out the forms at orientation seemed to have to search and shuffle through a lot of files on a table to find my forms. I remember thinking how stupid to have orientation on the top floor where new people have to go past all the other people working rather than on the first floor.

01/16/94 - The Chauffeur in the Limo (dream)

Very restful night and once again I dream. This time I am outside our house getting into a limo. I sit in the back seat facing the rear and the chauffeur gets in and sits opposite me. The chauffeur is me, he asks where my wife is and I say, "getting ready she'll be out in a minute." We wait for a long time, he asks if we should come back later. I say, "no I can wait here until she is ready." There is a wooden chest on the floor of the limo we don't notice what is in it but we discuss how it is constructed. I say that the wood seems thinner than the older chests that I remember from my youth. I say, "It seems that back then things were made to last forever but now you never know how long anything will last." The chauffeur says, "but you continue to wait?" I say, "I must you know, I must." I wake up.

01/22/94 - My Goddess Comes to Me (dream)

It is consummated. For the third day in a row I have erotic dreams. Unlike the three of the last two days in which my partner was Jean and we never come to completion this woman is a goddess, she is perfect in every way. I lay there naked as she tantalizes me in ways I have never been aroused before. Her tongue is hot in my mouth, her kiss causes me to burn in my loins. She softly kisses and caresses my body. I am so fully aroused that I burn all over, the same intense heat that I felt in my earlier fire dream. She puts her breasts in my face and I suckle from her. Her milk runs hot down my throat and arouses me ever more. I am at a state of ecstasy that I have never felt before. I consume all her milk from her breasts and feel very much loved. She moves my hands to her breasts and I feel her perfection. She guides my hands over her body to allow me to sense her even more. I have never felt such warmth emanate from a woman's body as I do at this time. Wherever I touch her she seems to tremble with excitement and glow with a deep inner warmth. She once again puts her breasts in my mouth then slowly moves her body over my lips, my tongue tastes the sweetness of her skin, she spreads her legs across my head and pulls me into her hot and moist body. I perform oral sex on her and she achieves a very powerful orgasm. I feel her whole-body quake with excitement as I satisfy her again and again. She then takes my penis into her hands and gently caresses me until I am feeling as though I will explode but I don't, I want more. She takes me into her mouth and brings my state of ecstasy even higher. She stops before I achieve orgasm and starts kissing me again deep and thrusting. She nuzzles my face in her bosom and finally mounts me and takes my penis into her body. She uses her body in ways that I cannot describe. I have an orgasm so powerful that I feel I am going to burst. The release is great and her body melts into mine and I feel more completely satisfied than I have ever felt in my life. She holds me so tight that her skin starts to burn against mine. One bodies merge and she is gone but I feel her within me gently caressing my very soul. I am at great peace within. I awake this morning warm and moist relaxed beyond belief. I seem giddy as a schoolgirl when I say Good Morning to Jean. Life is great.

01/23/94 - Jean's Hand in Marriage (dream)

I dream I am asking Jean's dad for her hand in marriage because it is the proper thing to do. Her dad is Jack and he says he'll agree with whatever Jean decides. Jean is unsure because she does not know if she can give up her father's love and care and move into a new relationship, she needs time to make up her mind. Once again, I am asked to wait, and I ask God why do I always have to wait. I do not get an answer. I wake up confused.

"The Road Less Traveled"
Problems I see in myself:

-I am always referring to Jean as "My bride" throughout our marriage. This may have hampered the natural growth process of our relationship. It was my failed attempt to keep the idyllic romantic love a constant rather than a basic building block for a deeper more binding love.

-Constantly denying my anger during our relationship in fear that if my anger was shown Jean would leave me. Healthy relationships become strengthened when anger (expressed but controlled) generates better understanding of needs, feelings and emotional boundaries.

Comments from the text:

p. 118 Couples sooner or later fall out of love, and it is at the moment when the mating instinct has run its course that the opportunity for genuine love begins.

p. 128 "We've been married 29 years and I never knew that about you before." When this occurs, we know that growth in the marriage has begun.
Jean and I have explored more and more each other's inner selves and have learned much about each other. Sometimes the learning is difficult. "Growth is painful."

p. 141 Couples cannot resolve in any healthy way the universal issues of marriage - dependency and independence, dominance and submission, freedom and fidelity, for example - without the security of knowing that the act of struggling over the issues will not itself destroy the relationship.

p. 166 The purpose and function of Lily (my wife) is to grow to be the most of which she is capable, not for my benefit but for her own and to the glory of God.
     - I must affirm this statement in my view of Jean.
     - A plus for me, I feel, is that I always supported Jean in any of her endeavors and never belittled her attempts at self-expression.
     - I only controlled where Jean relinquished control and constantly refused to accept control back.

p. 167 - 168   is significant.

p. 178 Any genuinely loving relationship is one of mutual psychotherapy. "How can I be a good friend, father, husband or son unless I take the opportunities that are available to attempt, with whatever artistry I command, to teach my beloved what I know and give whatever assistance is in my power to give to his or her personal journeys of spiritual growth?

Note to myself: I should look upon the last several months of emptiness on the part of Jean's love for me as a great opportunity for personal and spiritual growth. The loneliness and pain have caused me to perform much needed self-examination and behavioral adjustment. I owe Jean a great deal of thanks for being an instrument of my growth. I applaud her tenacity and strength.

Inner Work

01/24/94 - I Feel My Mistress Caress Me (active imagination)

I am very confused, many thoughts running through my mind in my dreams. This soft loving voice inside says, "It's OK, I'm here, let go, let me help." I start to go into a deep warm sleep then I become afraid, I cry out for Mommy but she's not there. I am awakened by Jean while in heavy sobs crying for my mother. My anguish over my mother's death a year ago is extremely painful. I am angry that she was not there for my birthday and died without saying goodbye. Jean asks how I am and I tell her I'm OK. I am because lately even while wide awake I can feel my mistress caress me and call to me. I know that she will always be there for me with total unconditional love because she is a very real and integral part of me. She makes me feel so warm and peaceful inside. I love her with my very soul.

01/25/94 - On a Jury (dream & analysis)

A very disturbing dream. I cannot remember many details only bits and pieces. On a jury, don't know what the trial is about at all. Eating at a large table with people. An enormous amount of food on the table. Am watching films of a man stripped naked and bound to some kind of fixture. Another man, tall and obviously in charge is parading around like a king. He brings in a beautiful woman who tantalizes the bound man. There is a connection between the two either they are married, engaged or in a relationship. As soon as the bound man shows any signs of excitement his handlers cause him great pain in the genitals. They seem to have a thong or strap attached to the man's penis and they yank it whenever he gets excited. The man in charge constantly laughs at the man's pain and keeps repeating the cycle of excitement and punishment. I awake in tears, crying for myself and my failures.

ANALYSIS:I reviewed this dream in depth with Bob Stoudt and identified the components as they related to me. The trial was in reality my inner struggle with the film I watched my inner view of myself. I identified most strongly with the person being tortured by his oppressors. I was strongly repulsed by the man in charge whom I described as possibly a Nazi or similar negative persona. Bob said it was good that I did not identify with the negative image as all images in dream work are parts of the self both good and bad. It is healthy to address these components of our inner self and accept each component for its strengths and weaknesses. I am fully aware of my inner struggle through this dream. It seems that inwardly I am confronting my external problems and resolving them through dreams. This allows me more freedom of expression in my daily life and the ability to overcome great pain. My personal growth is very difficult and painful but very fulfilling. I know I am struggling with great changes within and that the end result will be a stronger, healthier and more acceptable me. I am strong!

01/29/94 - The Invisible Partners

Yesterday Bob suggested I read this book to better understand what I am going through. Jean borrowed it from Jack. My appetite for knowledge seems voracious as I consumed this book in one day. I now understand the meaning of my pain. It is definitely great growth. I know why Bob said he hopes to keep Jean and I together long enough to complete this process. Seventeen years ago, we projected ourselves upon each other and a great bond of the unconscious collective occurred, for many years our inner selves enjoyed the external company of our projections. My struggle with the outer world caused great loneliness for both our inner selves and caused Jean to withdraw her projection into herself and allowed her to experience the great growth she is now enjoying. She then began her relationship with Jack and pushed my projection away from her putting me in great emotional stress. This stress was <u>finally</u> allowed by me to foster growth within and I feel great about it all. The book explains how through our mutual understanding of our individual inner process we both can and will grow spiritually. I finally believe now more than ever that Jean and I are meant to be and grow together forever. This gift from God should not be put aside for external wants and desires or fantasies put in front of us by our inner selves to cloud our judgement. We must both take hold of this great opportunity for growth and, with help from Bob to guide us through the process, develop into the separate individuals we are with the ultimate connectivity of our souls a goal.

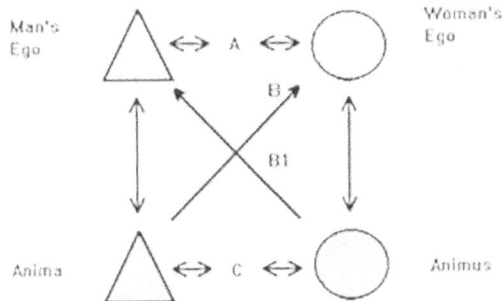

Anima & Animus

27

Inner Work

01/30/94 - A Request for My Old Poetry

I discussed with Jean my understanding of yesterday's reading and was not rebuked for my thoughts. I asked her for the poems I wrote to her in 1976 to review to better appreciate the feelings I had then and how they relate to now. I have reread them and am amazed at how deep and spiritual our attraction was then and how we must be truly blessed by God for having found each other. We must communicate more and build on this great gift of grace God has given us. We are the epitome of the rejoining of the anima and animus. We fill each other's souls with strength and love. Thank you, God, for the recent separateness we have experienced. I am learning and growing daily. I feel greatly loved by my mistress and my bond with Jean is acceptable to her. We must progress.

01/30/94 - Hand tilling a Field (dream)

My dream this morning: In a large field. Jean is at one end of a table full of starter plants preparing them to plant them in the field. I am hand tilling the field, removing large rocks and stones, turning the rich black soil with a shovel, rake and hoe. I am being encouraged by another woman who is beside me watching how well I clear the field. She constantly tells me I am doing well, the soil looks great, it is just the right consistency, be patient you have much more work to do. I am working toward Jean from the opposite side of the field. Whenever I check my progress, the woman next to me speaks soft words of encouragement, when I look over to Jean, she smiles approvingly then continues to prepare the seedlings for planting. I wake up while still working.

Inner Work

02/05/94 - A Pure White Vision of My Mistress (dream or active imagination)

Very restful night. I know I dreamed but it did not stay with me. Jean and I awake and just lay there in bed. She puts her hand on my chest and pats me gently. I hold her hand in my hands and feel her warmth against my chest. I flush of warmth goes over me and I fell at peace. I do not proceed to exaggerate the moment I just enjoy the inner peace. After a while she moves her hand and I place my arm next to her head she lays her arm on mine and I half sleep and day dream. As I close my eyes, I see pure white the harder I close them the whiter the white gets till it seems to glare. I see my mistress all dressed in white, she beckons to me and I feel very relaxed and at peace with everything. We do not touch only mentally communicate, somehow the scene changes and I am at the birth of my latest granddaughter Jacklyn. I once again feel the absolute joy of her birth. The scene changes again and I am observing my first granddaughter's birth. Ashley was born by C section. I do not see the actual operation, but I feel a great joy of birth. Once again, the scene changes and my wife is giving birth to our youngest son Anthony. This birth is evermore joyous than the previous scenes. I am very much at peace. The scene changes a last time and I watch the birth of my first son Michael. The process of rebirth is complete at each scene I was very much aware of my daughter's and wife's labor pains and felt the relief of birth and a deep flush of happiness. I returned to the area of bright white and felt much at peace. Both of my hands tingled with numbness as I awoke from my dream. Jean lat there beside me softly breathing. The world is looking brighter every day.

29

Inner Work

02/06/94 - My Oak Tree Dream

Fragment of a dream: Climbing a large tree to bend its boughs toward the ground to pick up a container. The container is for use at church. Pastor Barr is there. We are setting up for something, Chuck Kneuple is wondering how to light the oven and where it is. He is told to move a panel up. The oven is there but he does not know how to light it. I show him how to open the bottom he holds a match and I turn on the gas and the oven lights.

7 P.M.: Severe anxiety attack. Jack called at 6 to say he and Jean were stopping for dinner then come home in a couple of hours. I was not really positive in my response, I wish Jean would spend some quality time with me. My inner struggle is becoming very difficult. I need help desperately. Waiting for Bob to return my call.

NOTE: Bill Jumper called at 7:30 and we talked for hours.

02/16/94 - At My Own Funeral - Randy Barr & Train Engine (2 dreams)

Yesterday was hell. I talked with Jean and she said that she loved Jack and wanted to be with him from now on. I am crushed Thursday's meeting should be mostly a discussion on our next steps. I talked with Pastor Barr last night. Randy was very helpful in calming me down emotionally and he said he would be there for me. This morning Jean woke me from a nightmare and held me close to help me through it. I dreamed I was at my own viewing for my funeral. It was closed casket at Jean's request. Jean and jack are arm in arm at the casket and they say, "Now we can go on with our lives without his interference." I am alive inside the casket, I keep beating on the inside of the cover yelling "I am not dead yet let me out, please don't leave me here alone!!" No one can hear me. Everyone who stops at the casket says the same thing "At least he won't be able to run my life anymore." I watch as they put the casket into the hearse. I am now sobbing uncontrollably inside saying "No, no, please let me live." As they lower the casket into the ground. Jean wakes me up and asks if I am awake or dreaming. God she can comfort me when I feel bad to hold onto her calms me so much. I fall back to sleep and dream once again this time I am at St. Timothy's and Randy is driving a diesel train engine through the parking lot. One of Joan Appleton Jones' sons runs in front and is ran over. Randy and I look where he was and see his mangled body and we weep over his death and pray for his family to handle their grief. My back and chest muscles have been tight and painful all day. It is an effort to move without pain.

Inner Work

02/20/94 - Renewal of Wedding Vows (dream)

A good night's sleep and a fantastic dream. Our granddaughter's christening was beautiful full of love, family and warmth. Jean and I enjoy the warmth of our family's love and we embrace without strain or stress. It is suddenly our 17th wedding anniversary. We are at Penbrook with all our children, Jack, Sara, Char and Jim. Bob is presiding over a ceremony of renewal of our wedding vows. Jack escorts Jean to the altar to give her away then steps beside me as best man. The ceremony is very emotional. Sara is by Jean's side as matron of honor and Jack's daughters, Renee and Lee Ann are bridesmaids, Michael, Anthony, Cheech and Scot are ushers. There is great celebration as Jean and I commit ourselves to each other once again for life and the words of our voices ring loudly through the church. After the ceremony Jack comes to me and embraces me and says, "Can you forgive Jean and I for the pain we put you through? We are both very proud of your growth process and the only way you would see is if you were shocked into it. We love you and I wish you both the best in the future. I hope we can still remain friends." I am overwhelmed with joy for the return of my wife's love and our marriage. I tell Jack, "I have always liked you and never understood why you were taking Jean away. But I thank you for helping to start my growth. I will always love you as a member of our family and hope you will always be there for Jean and I when we need you. I am sorry for my anger at you these past few months, but I could not bear to lose the one person that I committed my life to!" I embrace Jack with a great hug and tell him I love him, forgive him and thank him for my new life. We both cry tears of happiness and I pull Jean to my side and embrace her and kiss her long and lovingly and everyone is happy for us. jean and I leave the church for an afternoon of rebirth. Jean and I look at each other once again with the love that seems to have eluded us these past few years. I feel a joy within my soul that I have never felt before as if for the first time in my life I finally understand what love really means. I awake with a smile on my face and come downstairs to write. It is 5 A.M. on the Sunday of the christening.

31

Inner Work

02/23/94 - Trolley Bridge Across a Chasm (dream)

Two lane trolley bridge across a chasm. Always misty, trolley always drive back and forth regularly with headlight on. One side is a town where I talk with a child searching for her father who seems to have disappeared on the other side. Other side is like a home for adults or a camp or something, cabins with four suites in each. I seem to always go to the same cabin as if I know he will be there I seem also to know which of the four rooms is his. I am searching the drawers in the room

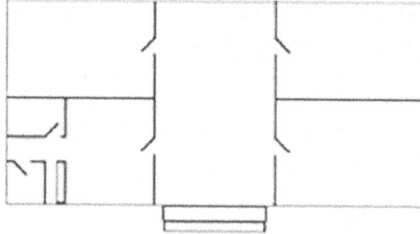

for a bottle of Scotch, he likes Scotch you know. I meet an old man each time I come to the cabin who says, "He's not gone really, he'll be back soon you will just have to wait." Everyone seems to have an Irish accent. I travel back and forth from the village to the camp many times. Each time I talk to the young girl in the village and give her hope. I always am searching when I return to the camp. The last time in the village she introduces me to the old man who was always at the camp and he says, "He's there now you know." I go to the bridge and neither trolley is running for a while. I walk across the bridge myself. It is a precarious journey, constantly watching for the headlight of a trolley so as to figure how to get out of its way. The bridge is slippery from the mist and footing is difficult. The bridge is very old and needs repair. I noticed that the roads in town were potholed. I finally reach the other side and the old man is waiting for me. "He's around now you know." I comment to him about the roads in town and the precarious walk I had across the bridge. He walks with me to the cabin and once again I search each room for that special bottle of Scotch. I find what seem to be small airline bottles of liquor in one room but no Scotch. I am worried that the other room occupants will be angry with me for looking through their things to find the drink for the little girl's father, but the old man tells me not to worry, "Everyone here understands and loves each other." I continue my search and find an excellent bottle of Scotch in one of the rooms. I never meet anyone in the camp though I seemed to notice them each time I enter. No one other than the old man ever speaks to me there. I sit down in my room in the cabin and pour myself a nice shot of Scotch. I slowly sip and enjoy the perfect flavor and look around the room. I realize that the Scotch was for me and that I was the person I was searching for in my dream that's why the old man said,

32

"He's here now you know." How many times had I taken the trolleys back and forth to give the little girl at the village hope before I crossed the bridge alone, the hard way, on slippery footing to find her father when all along it was me who I was searching for. I step out of the cabin and notice how beautiful the day is, the mist seems to have gone and the village streets are in perfect shape. Wait a minute the village is right outside my cabin door, the bridge I can finally see is merely a short footbridge crossing over a creek. There are no trolleys anywhere to be seen only people who seem exceedingly happy and full of life. Everything is so beautiful here I am at great peace. I have found myself and I like who I am.

02/23/94 - I Reread My Dreams (dreamwork)

I have reread my dream and am taking a break from work. I am accessing my situation in life and my real needs, wants and desires. The intro to "Inner Work" by Robert A. Johnson set the groundwork for last night's dream and my ability to so clearly transcribe it to paper. I am very much at peace today. I know that I still love Jean very much but that I do not want her love back as it was before as I have been hoping for these past months. My soul helped me select the proper anniversary card the other day but until this morning I was not fully aware of its meaning. I really want to begin anew with Jean if possible to start a new life full of loving, caring and sharing with a much more open relationship that allows room for everyone, me, Jean, the family, our extended families (including Jack), all our friends and associates. I want to express the inner love I feel to everyone I come in contact with. It is great to be alive and the world can kiss my ass if it wants to try to dampen my spirits. God is with me in my soul and no one or nothing can change that ever again.

02/26/94 - At a Military Hangar (dream & analysis)

At a military hangar. Marines are working on aircraft. I am in dress blues with sergeant stripes everyone else is in utilities. I am not wearing the proper rank. I take off the uniform and remove the stripes and insignia. A woman Marine is lining up the troops for marching. I am told to go change into my fatigues. I go to the men's locker and change. When at the drill area I take over for the woman Marine marching the troops. They weren't in step very well and I stopped them to remind them that they were Marines and should look sharp. We started marching again and this time they looked very sharp I sounded like a DI calling cadence. After marching four of them who seemed to be my friends were outside the hanger with me. I was reprimanding them for their attitude, but they just laughed and went on having fun. They finally stopped long enough to listen to me and I heard them tell me to lighten up and don't be so rigid about everything "you're only a paean like us you know, relax." We ran into the field nearby to have fun. We are no longer in uniform but in casual clothes walking outside the base. We know that we do not have to return there ever again. We are full of happiness, me and my four friends.

NOTES:

Military base -regimented life, forced lifestyle, uniforms, cold environment.
Sergeant uniform - authority figure, controlling person, always right even when wrong.
Woman leader -equal to me, soft-spoken but firm.
Troops - disorganized group of misfits, basic give-a-shit attitude, rejects regimentation, would rather switch than fight, want out of the regimen.
Me as DI - strong leader, able to get troops to organize, upset with poor marching, could not change friends' attitudes, joined them in the outside world.
Four friends - 3 men and a woman, happy-go-lucky types, full of life, rejected the regimentation, smiling as we left the base to freedom. The woman seemed to lead us all as we left.

02/27/94 - A Long Journey Over Mountains (dream & analysis)

Another dream of a long journey. I am walking over mountains, it is raining heavily. As I reach a peak, I see a beautiful panoramic view of the whole mountain range. The sky is clear and bright, and the majesty of the mountains is awe inspiring and breathtaking. I can see my destination in the distance and that the rest of my journey will also be difficult with heavy rains. I take in the beauty of the moment as if using it for inner strength and start down the mountain to finish my journey. The rest of my journey is difficult with poor footing due to the heavy rains and mud, but I come to mountain tops for refreshment and peaceful beauty several times. Each time the beauty is overwhelming and fills me with peace and strength. I finish my journey and make calls to family and friends to let them know that I made it OK. I go to my house and Jean and the kids are there to greet me, happy to see I returned from my long journey safely. Jean beckons me to the bedroom and locks the door saying, "I want you, I have missed you so much, make love to me now." I turn the light switch off, but the light stays on. I unscrew the bulb but there is still light coming from the ceiling. I cannot darken the room. Jean is naked beckoning to me, so I quit trying to put out the lights and go to her. She kisses me passionately and pulls my head into her bosom for me to suckle. It feels so good to hold her and have her want me again. We hear a noise and there are the faces of our two sons and two of Mike's friends at the window watching us with glee. I am afraid Jean will stop if we are being watched but she says, "Ignore them, make love to me, I want you now!" I awake embraced in the warmth of her love.

NOTES:

Mountain tops -the top of the world, as near to God as humanly possible, the panoramic beauty is a view of God's majesty and vastness. Above the bad weather - trials and tribulations of day to day life. Peaceful, serene, fulfilling, source of strength and energy.

Rain & mud - difficult road to travel, life's hardships and burdens. Uneasy footing and struggling to reach a final destination.

Home town -journey's end, a safe place of refuge and peace. My inner space, my soul's domain, in touch (home safe calls) with my many selves. The place to be, HOME!

My house - my castle where my soul and I live in peace and harmony.

Jean / bedroom - Jean is my soulmate, she fills me with unquenchable love and emotion. The light in the bedroom that will not be turned off is God's love for me and a blessing to our bond in bed.

4 boys at window - young, inquisitive children, very happy to see our bonding and our mutual love. Very approving.

02/27/94 - A Review of the Past Week

This has been a very peaceful week. Jean and I have had lunch together every day. We have nice conversations, no animosity. I am getting much better at listening, I think. Saturday morning, we both discussed the dreams we had and after brushing her teeth Jean came to the bed and sat down right next to me. I instinctively pulled her to me and gave her a hug, kissed the back of her neck and told her I loved her. She hugged me back and thanked me for the hug. It felt so good. Jack came at 8:00 to pick Jean up as they were helping Sara (his sister) move. As she left she called me honey and kissed me goodbye on the lips. At 2 PM she called from the Colonial Park Diner for me to pick her up, so she could make it to Tony's Blue and Gold Dinner with us. I ate with her at the diner then we headed home. I placed my hand on her leg as we started to drive, and she did not remove it as usual. She let me softly hold onto her thigh the whole journey. We talked at home before leaving for the dinner, she was looking out the French doors of the family room at the back yard and was commenting on the beauty of the day. I came up from behind her and put my arms around her waist and looked out with her. She did not reject my embrace as she usually did. We looked out at the sunny day for a moment then she went up to get ready. She thanked me several times for "rescuing her". At the dinner she laughed with me and hugged me from behind as we watched the show on stage. It was very peaceful and warm. I did NOT push the feeling I was having. I inwardly enjoyed the good times and I hope for more. We both slept well last night and we both dreamed. The alarm went off and I pulled Jean to me for a hug and she put her arm around me and rested her head on my chest. I caressed the small of her back as we lay there embracing and enjoyed the softness of her skin. Once again, I kept my feelings in and enjoyed the peace they brought to me. Jack is picking her up for breakfast and church and possibly lunch but that's OK. She says she will not be late like she used to be, and I say OK. I am doing much better at keeping my thoughts inside and waiting for the natural flow to occur. Change and growth is slow and painful but very rewarding.

02/28/94 - At A Mall Applying for Work (dream)

Strange dream, I awake sad on the verge of tears missing mom. I am at a Mall applying for a job. I meet the interviewer who seems to care less about me. I am with someone, perhaps my father, I turn in applications for three different positions. I ask dad if I filled out the one for the position I really wanted correctly then say, "It doesn't matter since I already work here, I am just looking at these other positions for a change of work. They should know who I am from my records." I am taking copies of my paperwork with me and I ask for a box to put them in, I seem to be at my dad's home in the foyer. My aunt tells my cousin to get me a shoe box from the closet. He brings out a pile of boxes and gives me the bottom one to use. I notice I am putting toys (cars and such) in a pile to put in the box. I seem to be a child now getting ready to leave and am using the box to store my toys. I open the box (a bowling shoe box). In the box are papers. I pick up the top sheet and it is an old bowling score sheet. I ask if anyone needs it and my aunt says, "No Frankie throw it out but make sure nothing else is in the box that is important." As I sift through the contents of the box I notice a pair of baby shoes, pictures of my mom holding a new baby boy, I also notice letters from mom and dad to each other while he was in Korea when I was very young. God they loved each other and missed being together while dad was away. I show the contents to dad and we both become sad at mom's death, I am myself again a grown man talking with dad and Aunt Ethyl about mom.

02/28/94 - I Talk with My Goddess (active imagination)

Before going to bed this evening Jean and I discussed her session with Bob then I went down to let the dogs out one last time. While waiting for them to finish I talked to my goddess, she was trying to get me angry about Jean. I told her I loved her and Jean both and that she was very special and important to me and to not get angry that Jean rejected her projection last year because it allowed me to find her and join with her and I won't abandon her.

03/01/94 - A Ritual to Affirm My Dream

Last night I performed a ritual to affirm my dreams of earlier days as suggested in "Inner Work." After my chasm dream, I purchased a bottle of 15-year-old "Pinch" scotch, my favorite. Saturday, I opened the bottle to enjoy a shot of it on the rocks. Last night I decided that a proper ritual to connect my dream work with my daily external conscious life was to pour the bottle down the drain as a symbol of completeness, a task finished. I poured the bottle down the drain and rinsed it out and returned it to its box. I plan to keep this as a reminder of my ritual.

03/02/94 - Returning to a Place from The Past (dream & analysis)

Last night I had an interesting dream. I was returning to a place from my past. I walked into the building and everything inside was in ruin, I think I used to play on stage at the bar in this building. It seemed to have been a museum also with anything relating to my past destroyed. I am escorted through the rubble by the proprietress. The only thing I find unbroken is a harmonica which she gives to me to keep. It seems brand new and in perfect shape, odd among a room of rubble. I notice a new wing being worked on. It seems to be a craft museum or something. I ask the proprietress when it will be ready, and she says, "Very soon would you like to take a look inside?" I join her and walk through the rubble into the new wing, it is a beautiful room in perfect order with much art and Indian Craft work on display. As we enter the room, we seem to be in a church immediately. We are sitting in a pew together. I start to daydream during the service and I write down my dream. I dream about Mexico and its ancient ruins. We receive communion together. The priest gives us the bread in our hands, we partake of the bread and I notice we both have a huge piece left in our hand. The priest says, "Take it with you for nourishment." We return to our pew and the man who was sitting next to me was reading my dream notes. He had his own notes and was comparing them to mine. He says, "Isn't it strange we both wrote about Mexico?" I notice Jean and friends in the next pew and I mention the common dreams and Jean says, "That's interesting." I turn around to sit facing the altar and the man points out the new wing to the left that is just completed. He says, "I can't wait for the choir to use the new loft over there, it will sound beautiful, you will join us and sing, won't you?" I wake up and start to write. I noticed that the new wing completed the fourth part of the cross shape of the building. The church is now balanced. From the priest's perspective the new wing is on his right hand.

Craft room - American Indian and Mexican artifacts, beautiful serape as we look in. Indian pottery, headdresses, jewelry, fantastic peace pipe with 12 eagle feathers on stem. Old Spanish or Mexican clay figures and pottery. All in excellent condition as if carefully uncovered during dig.

03/03/94 - Kitchen Floor Covered in Brown Rice (dream)

Strange night, Jean awakens about 4 AM and sits up. I ask her if she's OK she says, "No!" She tries to lay down to sleep but can't get comfortable and complains "I wish I could just sleep in my bed without it moving or vibrating." She always seems to blame me for the bed vibrating. I am lying perfectly still and feel no motion. This has occurred often lately. I go back to sleep and then awake sharply from a dream. I am in the kitchen and the floor is covered with cooked brown rice. I blame the dogs for pulling plates off the counters to scatter the food. The rice is 2 - 3 inches thick. I am sweeping it into piles, moving chairs and complaining "Why can't one of you help me clean this mess up?" I finally throw my hands up and say, "Fuck it this is too much!" I wake up.

03/03/94 - The Choir Master (dream)

I fall back to sleep finally. The alarm wakes me again from a dream. This time I am talking with a choir master, he is asking me what musical instruments I play, and can I sing the other voices or only bass. I am upset with his seemingly adamant stance that one must play several instruments and sing all voices to join or be at least accepted. I am walking around a square black table with a woman member of the choir and telling her of the absurd request he made of me. As I walk around the table with her, I am polishing the edges of the table as I finish circling and polishing I stop at a smaller square table and polish it also. I am still upset about the director's request. I am searching through my choir folder for today's anthem as the other members are lining up to enter church to sing. I am having trouble finding the music. I dump the contents of my folder on the large table and start looking through the papers. My left lens falls out of my glasses and the screw is there beside it. I ask the director for help repairing my glasses, so I can join the others to sing. He comes over to help repair my glasses and I wake up.

03/05/94 - Committing Hari Kari (dream)

Dream or Active Imagination not sure which, it seemed so real. At Penbrook on Sunday, Sunday school session, ask Bob for permission to use stage for a ritual. Bob says OK. I am wearing Japanese garb. Sequence repeats several times until done right. Preparing to commit Hari Kari on stage. Start with small kitchen knife, then a Ginzu and Finally dad's Marine Corps officer's sword. Final time I had a Tami mat to place on floor, a small bowl of rice and another of salt, a carafe of Saki and a small earthen goblet. I take the rice and salt then scatter some of each in a circle around me, I drink the goblet of Saki. I pray loudly for forgiveness then unsheathe the sword and prepare to disembowel myself. I awake abruptly, hot, sweating profusely, definitely shaken. I am writing this the next day and upon writing the previous sentence my hands shake and I get goose bumps all over my body.

03/09/94 - St. Exupery

"A rock pile ceases to be a rock pile the moment a single man contemplates it, bearing within him the image of a cathedral."
St. Exupery

03/10/94 - Electronics Lab (dream)

In an electronics lab repairing optical equipment. System will not work, I apprize the problem point out the failing component replace it and the system comes up. I show others how it works controlling the light source with an interference filter. I seem to be the lead engineer, my knowledge is revered by the others. I drive away and as in a previous dream road work seems to be blocking the way, but I am allowed to pass by everyone else. Someone has a tire problem, I have the exact tires needed to fix it for them. I walk around a stopped truck in the snow it too has a flat tire and I seem to have the proper replacement in my hands. It is cold, snowy and damp the side of the road. I wake up by Jean touching my cheek to ask me if I'm OK, I say I'm cold. She allows me to embrace her hand on my chest until the alarm goes off.

03/11/94 - *Superheroes, Supervillians and Julian's Birth (dream)*

Rack of comic books, all are about different Superheroes and Supervillians. Each comic has an exact reverse version, if one has a good guy in red and dark blue another has a bad guy in dark blue and red. Searching for a specific one. Others helping look comment on action scenes on covers. A child is being born, I tightly embrace the woman to feel the contractions and hear the heartbeat of the child. I watch the contractions tighten her body as delivery starts. It is a boy and we are trying to name the child, names are suggested Jeffery or Julian seem to be the choices most mentioned. Jeffery is discounted because of another child who has that name that is difficult. The mother talks of her dream before labor and she was looking for a comic book also and there was a man in all black observing her search, I said, "I saw the same man in my comic store he almost looked 2 dimensional like a shadow. She agreed that in her dream he appeared the same. The shadow person we both agreed must have been our dark side helping us find what we wanted. The shadow person was with both of us watching us search and seemed pleased that we settled on Julian as the name for our child. He said, "Julian is a name of kings you know!" We both agreed and then I woke up. When I woke up this dream was the most vivid that I can remember. I felt as if I was not even asleep through it. I was exhausted from the labor and delivery as if I were the woman giving birth. The child was perfect and smiled as he was delivered. I do not recall the umbilical cord being cut because the child was perfectly clean when delivered, no mess, no blood, just a beautiful child. There were the four of us me, the woman, the male child and the shadow. It is 4 AM.

Inner Work

03/14/94 - "Phaedra, I am called Phaedra!" (active imagination)

Lunch with Jean is very enjoyable. Our conversations now tend to be more about inner growth and spirituality. Jean feels a burning deep inside when she asks a question inward using her name. I think her depth of inner consciousness is expanding and I am enjoying her sharing these realizations with me. I know the feeling she described I have similar feelings when I talk to my goddess. On the way back from lunch I wondered about the name of the little girl in my chasm dream, all of a sudden, I was beside her where she was sitting near the trolley bridge at the beginning of my dream. I asked her what her name was, and she looked up at me shyly and said in a soft children's little girl voice "Phaedra, I am called Phaedra!" I thought how beautiful her name was and chills ran up my spine to my fingertips and my face felt warm from within. I felt very much at inner peace.

03/15/94 - Flying on the Outside of a Plane (dream)

Flying in a plane. My seat seems to be on the outside I have to hold on to the back of the seat to keep from falling at first then I realize I won't fall out. The sky is beautiful up here, blue and bright with friendly fluffy white clouds and a brilliant sun. I am carrying in my arms an important package.

NOTE: I seem to be able to call to Phaedra at will and hear her respond to me. I ask for her support and strength in my processes and she assures me she is there for me.

03/18/94 - Jean and I with Bob

I felt hopelessness while listening to Jean discuss the people who she wasn't good enough for, her dad, Uncle Bill, Ronnie. I feel I am paying the price for their sins. Now that Jack has entered the picture, she finally has a male from her immediate family that fills her emotional needs and I am left out in the cold.

03/19/94 - Basement of New Building (fire dream & analysis)

Basement of new building. Fire causing intense heat blocks escape route to the left through tunnel. Window opening behind us, wide trench outside, I look up, construction material precariously hanging above. Call for help. Someone throws a wet blanket through window then tries to put plank from ground level to window. Construction material falls

41

and blocks window. Tunnel only way out. Intense heat. Young boy is wrapped in wet blanket to shield from heat. Using child in blanket as a shield I push into tunnel repelled by force of inferno. Contemplate what to do, realize that fiery tunnel is only way out and the child in the blanket may have to perish while being a shield. Finally take a deep breath and run into tunnel on left with child as shield. Heat is white hot as we run into tunnel. I am holding child in front of me. An opening to the left is reached and I jump to the left for safety. The child in the blanket seems to evaporate in the white heat as they protect me from harm and I escape. The fire was started earlier in my dream to block the way from some other evil people getting to us. The child was not always there he just seemed to appear when I realized the flaming tunnel was the only way out and I would surely perish if I entered the tunnel without something to block the intense heat. The wet blanket around the child was my shield. He did not ignite and burn up in the flames as he protected me only evaporated into white light that completely blocked the intense heat as I escaped.

Basement area Dirt floor, newly dug, red clay, walls did not seem solid just deep black borders that could not be crossed, maybe even shadowy. Window was just an opening in the wall behind me an easy way out if the building material hadn't collapsed in front of it.

03/20/94 - The Journey Inward (dream)

As I journey deeper inward past my heart and towards my soul, I cross the Misty Mountains through an ageless pass to the emerald green valley in which resides my soul. A perpetual rainbow crosses the valley through the mist, there, beneath the highest point of its arch, lies a grassy knoll smothered in lilacs. In the center of the lilacs is an alabaster stand upon which a book as old as time itself sits written in God's own hand. As I leaf through the pages of my life, I search the glossary in the back for definitions. The definitions are images from God to guide me in my quest. As I read the words the images appear in my mind.

Beauty	The image of a goddess appears
Care, Comfort	My goddess's arms reach out as to embrace my soul.
Sweetness	My goddess's moist lips sparkle in the sunbeams.
Happiness	My goddess's eyes beam with joy
Love	My goddess's heart glows from within as her face beams with a warm smile of inner love.

Inner Work

Dear Jean,

I am asking Bob to read this letter for a reason. Lately anytime I talk to you it is taken as if I am trying to do something "TO" you. I did not start nor even continue the present rift between us. Our children today talked to you about their feelings. I did not tell them what to say. Renee and Lee Ann are adults and as such speak their own minds. <u>YOU</u> told them that Jack had asked you to marry him. Their response was less than positive. I reminded you that you have not even separated from me much less filed for divorce. You hugged me and said, "nothing has been decided." I asked if you knew how long it took in Pennsylvania to get a divorce and you said, "three months if no-fault" and I said, "two years if I don't agree." You were upset that I would not give you a no-fault and do that "TO" you. I feel that by making you wait the full two years that I would be doing that "FOR" you not to you because I love you very much and having read and studied about mid-life as I have. Borrowing books from Jack and Bob and buying many others I feel that I have a fairly good grasp on what is happening. We are both undergoing great inner changes and the end result will be both of us being very healthy. I am sorry that I cannot give you and Jack carte blanche with your future, but I will delay your gratification as long as I can to allow you to be given the space and time you need to reach the best possible decision for yourself. I do not hold any hope at this time that our marriage or for that matter our friendship can endure the deep pain you have inflicted upon me, but I keep praying and asking God to help me to be strong. I am very saddened by the pain you must be feeling and wish that I could change that but at this point I can only say that all that you feel and see happening "TO" you is a direct result of decisions and statements "YOU" have made or said. I no longer wish to be the dumping ground for your troubles. If your world is turning to shit, ask Jack why he is burying you in feces. I am not the cause nor the effect in your present life's trials and tribulations. The cause and effect is asking you to forsake not only our marriage but your whole family for his selfish desires. I have and will give you the space you need to find yourself. If after your search I am not to be a part of your life so be it, but at least find out for yourself. Ask Jack to give you the same dignity I have given you and to leave you alone long enough for you to resolve your inner conflicts. I love you very much and will be your support as long as you need it to help you get through this change. Please believe me when I say I love you: you are the best thing that ever happened to me. I am not sure that I was <u>ever</u> worthy of your love.

Inner Work

04/05/94 - Olympic Racing Team (dream)

Running, rollerblading or biking across country as a part of a team, Olympic I believe. Interviewed at one stop while dodging snow piles in streets. I predicted another storm in the next week or two of several inches. Another racer agrees with me. Observing country from above watching race progress from east to west in a zigzag pattern. Fireworks are exploding in the air at each stop across the country. At west coast city at end of journey. Golden uniformed team members swinging back and forth in rigging of a large sailing ship performing for a crowd below. I am one of the performers. Below a large American flag is stretched out and being dedicated to the team.

"Dear members, this flag is dedicated to all participants in the great competition ahead especially the men as this flag is a memorial to the little boy in me who died while being born. I feel a great emptiness and loss at his passing. Please divide this flag among yourselves and carry the pieces with you throughout your life as a symbol of a child who gave his all in his struggle. Thank you for the opportunity to be with you during this time of preparation as I will not be able to compete with you as my inner pain is too much to bear. I love all of you, but I must rest."

04/07/94 - Birth of a Butterfly

Last night at our session with Bob, Jean emerged from her cocoon, a beautiful butterfly, whole, healthy and ready to take wing. She pronounced that she did not need me to take care of her or protect her from herself or her decisions and that she wanted a divorce now, done and did. I thanked her for showing me her birth, applauded her strength and granted her the freedom she has struggled so hard for. I go on my retreat this weekend with sadness, happiness, pain, anxiety and searching. I look to God for answers in my life.

Inner Work

WERNERSVILLE RETREAT CENTER JOURNAL

04/08/94 - 8:20 PM – Arrival at Wernersville

Visited the Grotto and as I walked back to the Novitiate, I looked across the large green expanse in front of the building and saw the oak tree from my dream. Every branch was exactly as I saw it in my dream, the sight stopped me in my tracks, I knew this place before I ever arrived. I walked up to the tree and touched it and felt good inwardly. I met Rikki, a female Episcopal minister, she is older, wiser and friendly. I leave outside these gates my pain and sufferings of the past and open my heart to God's grace and love. Near the Grotto a small rabbit stood looking at me, I said, "Hello, I love you!" He did not run away. I ran through the green grass and jumped for joy at the beauty around me. I stretched out on the grass in the sunshine, spread my arms and drank in the sunshine. I thanked God for loving me and pledged my undying love and devotion to him.

04/09/94 7:45 AM – First Morning Observations

Slept poorly, anxiety over my marriage predominates my thoughts. God reminds me I am not perfect. I thank Him for His love and ask forgiveness for my sins.

9:00 AM - Walking and praying asking God's guidance.

Was reading Isaiah and felt I should revisit my choices of the past and my interpretation of recent events.

My struggle at midlife:

Maybe a recalling by God to my earlier vocation.

Jean's struggle:

God helping to sever our ties to free me for my vocation. She is a great mother and full of love.

Jack's presence in Jean's life:

God's replacement for me to help Jean and the family if I change vocations.

My dreams and poems:

God's words of direction and encouragement to fulfill my vocational needs.

10:45 AM - Meeting with Fr. Jack Barron

He recommends several scripture passages for me to read and contemplate the next couple of days. They prove most thought provoking and directional. I rewrite them here directed at me:

Inner Work

Isaiah 43: 1 - 7
> But now, thus says the Lord, who created you, O Frank,
>> and formed you, O Frank:
> Fear not, for I have redeemed you;
>> I have called you by name: you are mine.
> When you pass through the water, I will be with you;
>> in the rivers you shall not drown.
> When you walk through fire you shall not be burned;
>> the flames shall not consume you.
> For I am the Lord, your God,
>> the Holy One of Israel, your savior.
> I give Egypt as your ransom,
>> Ethiopia and Seba in return for you.
> Because you are precious in my eyes and glorious,
>> and because I love you.
> I give men in return for you and people
>> in exchange for your life.
> Fear not, for I am with you; from the east I will bring back
>> your descendants, from the west I will gather you.
> I will say to the north: Give them up!
>> and to the south: Hold not back!
> Bring back my sons from afar, and my daughters
>> from the ends of the earth:
> Frank who is named is mine, whom I created for my glory,
>> whom I formed and made.

Inner Work

Isaiah 55: 1 - 3

> Frank who is thirsty come to the water! You who have no money,
>> come, receive grain and eat;
>
> Come without paying and without cost,
>> drink wine and milk!
>
> Why spend your money for what is not bread;
>> your wages for what fails to satisfy?
>
> Heed me, and you shall eat well,
>> you shall delight in rich fare.
>
> Come to me heedfully, listen,
>> that you may have life.
>
> I will renew with you the everlasting covenant,
>> the benefits assured to David.

Isaiah 55: 8 – 13

> For my thoughts are not your thoughts,
>> nor are your ways my ways, says the Lord.
>
> As high as the heavens are above the earth, so high are my ways above
>> your ways and my thoughts above your thoughts.
>
> For just as from the heavens
>> the rain and snow come down
>
> And do not return there till they have watered the earth,
>> making it fertile and fruitful,
>
> Giving seed to him who sows
>> and bread to him who eats,
>
> So shall my word be
>> that goes forth from my mouth;
>
> It shall not return to me void, but shall do my will,
>> achieving the end for which I sent it.
>
> Yes, in joy you shall depart,
>> in peace you shall be brought back;
>
> Mountains and hills shall break out is song before you,
>> nd all the trees of the countryside shall clap their hands.
>
> In place of the thorn bush, the cypress shall grow,
>> instead of nettles, the myrtle,
>
> This shall be to the Lord's renown,
>> an everlasting imperishable sign.

Inner Work

1:00 PM – A Relaxing Massage

I scheduled myself for a massage to help relax my body. I could feel the tension leaving my body as the LPN's hands worked on my tired muscles. She asks me afterward if I have been feeling inner conflict as she felt another presence emanating from me as she massaged me as if someone were trying to communicate from within. I said that I have been doing inner work with a pastor and my dreams have been very dominant of late with many different persons in communication with me. I was amazed that someone could actually feel that presence emanating from me. She has been having vocational dreams for the past three or four years and is considering becoming a nun. This place is so peaceful and full of love. I am glad I came here for retreat and am sorry I must return to the world outside. Jane mentioned that she heard a name when she touched me, the name was Seth. I know no one named Seth so I looked in the Bible. there is only one Seth in the Bible. He is the third son of Adam and the first child to be the exact likeness of Adam according to Genesis. It is also from his lineage that Joseph, Christ's human father, is descended.

5:45 PM – Dinner in Silence

Dinner in silence is invigorating, people politely nod or smile at each other. The warmth felt without spoken words is phenomenal. God has gifted me with great love and grace this weekend. Father Jack Barron allowed me to receive Holy Communion today. I explained my position, divorced and remarried. He asked if I believed in the presence of our Lord in the bread and wine. I said, "With my whole heart." He said, "Join us at the altar, we do not punish here but welcome you to the Lord's supper." I felt great receiving the sacrament in a Catholic service once again. God loves me and I am happy. My complete retreat experience is written in prose in "Visions of God's Love"

Inner Work

04/10/94 – God Opens My Bible

God opened my Bible to Isaiah 9: 1 - 6 this morning and the words touched my very soul and filled me with grace and hope. I rewrote it directed at me.

> Frank who walked in darkness has
> > seen a great light;
>
> Upon he who dwelt in the land of gloom
> > a light has shone.
>
> You have brought him abundant joy
> > and great rejoicing,
>
> As he rejoices before you at the harvest,
> > as men make merry when dividing spoils.
>
> For the yoke that burdened him, the
> > pole on his shoulder
>
> And the rod of his taskmaster you have
> > smashed, as on the day of Midian.
>
> For every boot that trampled in battle, every
> > cloak rolled in blood, will be burned
> > as fuel for flames.
>
> For a child is born to us, a son is given us;
> > upon his shoulder dominion rests
>
> They name him Wonder-Counselor,
> > God-Hero, Father-Forever, Prince of Peace.
>
> His dominion is vast and forever peaceful,
> > Which he confirms and sustains
>
> By judgement and justice, both now and forever.

04/10/94   Visions of God's Love

Rolling hills bursting with the birth of spring
Birds singing softly in the shadows of dusk
God's gentle breezes wafting over us with love
A mighty oak with outstretched arms beckons
I lay calmly on a grassy knoll drinking in the sun
God's love pours warmly over me as I rest
A sleepless night contemplating life
Breakfast in silence brings peace to the soul
God's presence here permeates the very walls
A run through the field invigorates the spirit
The Grotto offers winter's snow and prayer
God touches my heart and I feel loved
My director's voice and words soothe me
A quiet lunch where smiles are shared

Inner Work

God gifts us all with inner peace
Holy Communion fills my soul with hope
Sharing peace with strangers creates a bond
God's grace flows from everyone into me
A wonderful massage to relax my body
Sharing dreams expands the experience
God's hand is felt in the gentle hands that touch me
More prayer and communion with God
Isaiah's words bring peace and enlightenment
God is my creator and God loves me forever
A return to the grassy knoll and quiet prayer
A vision in the clouds appears to me
God's hand has written in the clouds
I draw the vision on paper with pencil
It appears to be written in Hebrew

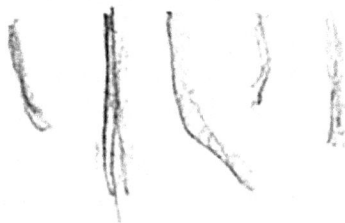

God help me find the meaning
Dinner is shared in silence with soft music playing
A young girl is seated across from me with sparkling eyes
God's gentleness glows from her smile
Silent prayer fills the void in my soul
Instead of sleep inner work is done
God has helped me through another difficult night
An early shower then a walk outside
Back to my knoll then a rosary at the Grotto
God is praised in song "He Leadeth Me"
Silent breakfast again with the young girl
Her eyes and smiles fill my soul with grace
God has put her there to show me His beauty
As she gifted me with her silent smiles
I gifted her with a letter of thanks and a poem
God's words written by me in "A Journey Inward"
A short nap refreshes the weary mind
A gentle rain begins, a walk is delayed
God is watering his lovely earth
I sit in tears in the Holy Spirit Chapel
Tears of loss for a love and a marriage
God holds me in His arms and comforts me

The rain stops, the birds start singing
A silent smile crosses my pained face
God has made me feel His love once again
A final nap then a recap with Fr. Jack Barron
With grace and understanding he blesses my journey
God placed me in the right place this weekend

I leave this retreat whole and thanking God.

04/16/94 - In Africa or some other jungle area (dream)

In Africa or some other jungle area. Journey to make but no mode of transportation except walking. A small train goes by but it is just an engine and coal car and not allowed to accept riders. I walk away then think how nice it would be if I had brought my car. Immediately I was driving an immaculate condition car from the 50's down a dirt road beside a beautiful river on the left of me and tall grassy plains to the right. I notice several huge crocodiles sitting on the river bank watching me pass by, they seem almost friendly. I remember an old song "Never smile at a crocodile, no you can't get friendly with a crocodile." so I keep moving on. The road is barely wide enough for one car but several times I meet an oncoming vehicle and there always seems to be a widening in the road as we meet so we can pass each other without stopping. I see many beautiful animals and birds on my journey. It is so beautiful and peaceful here. At the end of the road I leave my car and begin walking again. I am at a clearing with a beautiful pond off to my left and a small field to my right. There does not seem to be any way to leave this place once you get here. There are no paths leading away. I walk around the pond pondering the beauty of where I am and then a large fish swims to the edge of the pond and says, "Hello!" I stop and look at him and he is just smiling at me half out of the water and says, "Hello!" to me again. I remark about the beauty of this place and that I noticed a baseball backstop above on the hill but there was no way to get up there to play. The fish says, "Go play over there!" Then he jumps in the air in the direction of the green field on the other side of the pond and swims away. I walk over to the clearing and pick up the baseball and throw it to the young boy who is standing there. We play catch for a while then it seems that when I throw the ball it becomes attached to a large red elastic or rubber band and comes back at me fast but always stops just short of hitting me. I lay on a small child's bed to rest and assure the boy that my wife and my weight would not break his bed. I sit up and look around at the beauty of the area and feel great.

NOTE: The end of the journey area that I said there seemed no way to leave. It wasn't that I couldn't walk out if I wished only that I felt once

I got there, I was not supposed to leave and really didn't wish to leave.

04/16/94 – A Conversation with jack

I talked to Jack this morning and read him a letter I wrote to Jean concerning the past few months and Easter Sunday. We discussed our basic beliefs. He told me his base of belief was different than mine. He believes that as long as you feel in your heart that what you are doing is right then it is OK with God. I feel sad for Jack as he puts human feelings before God's guidance. I pray for his better understanding of God's teachings and wish him well in life. Mary Lou called this morning and we had a very nice talk. As I lay there on the bed talking with her of my weekend with God, I noticed sunlight reflecting from some water on the ground through the window. I told Mary Lou what I was seeing. The sun projected a cross on the ceiling as the water reflecting it must have been small enough to only cast a shadow of two panes of the window. The sunlight dances behind the cross like white flames glowing. I felt very much in touch with God as I watched the cross on the ceiling. My life is becoming fuller of God's love and grace every day. Jean is away this weekend on a journey to the shore. I hope God touches her as He touched me last weekend. I do not know where our lives are leading but I know that God is directing us down a path of discovery. Mary Lou said she and Jimmy noticed a change in me a year ago. She said I seemed humbler and I listened to people better. God is working in me and giving me bountiful grace. I must follow wherever He is leading me. I pray for His guidance in my journey.

04/19/94 - Sailing on a Beautiful 3 Masted Schooner (dream)

Sailing on a beautiful 3 masted schooner, white sails arching in the strong wind. We are sailing to a special destination, a black hole where Jean and I are going to get out of the ship and walk towards the center of the black hole to see what changes it will cause in us. We are not making this journey as mates only two individuals searching for themselves. I am being prepared for the walk each day with a staff of three people making me up, so I look proper for facing my challenge and with daily contemplation on my journey and the goal I am heading toward. I know that I will not face the final challenge at the black hole in this dream only prepare for it in future dreams. I take walks on the deck to enjoy the sun and breeze and pray for guidance.

04/20/94 - A RETURN TO WERNERSVILLE IS MADE

A return to Wernersville is made. I had to come back here this week to once again get in touch with God.
I arrived at 10 AM and checked in

Inner Work

04/21/94 – A Day of Contemplation

Prayer on my grassy knoll and a visit to my oak begins my visit.
Contemplative prayer in my room prepares me for union with God.
Mass and Eucharist Toshi presiding in the Holy Spirit Chapel.
We pray for peace and healing, Peace of God is warmly shared.
I enjoy lunch with friends and talk of our journeys with God.
I share my poems with Hobie (a novice)
A long walk to the little Grotto.
Four deer watch me patiently, then scurry away white tails erect.
A pheasant crows in the distance.
I walk the Stations of the Cross in the woods.
A rosary made of stone on the ground in a clearing.
Prayers are said at the statue of the Sacred Heart.
A short talk with Mom and Mary at the little Grotto.
Tears are shed.
The flowers abound jonquils, crocus, blue bells, clover, forsythia.
Trees are bursting with new born leaves.
Squirrels and birds dash and flit about.
A relaxing stroll to the lake where I sit and pray.
Two large turtles watch me write while they bask in the warm afternoon sun.
Goldfish gently glide beneath the cool waters, large beautiful goldfish one 2 to 3 feet long.
It is so peaceful here, a small sweat bee rests on my sleeve.
Powder blue butterflies dance in the pines.
A walk past St. Rene Goupil's shrine.
A shrine to the Madonna (Mary's Wall) is visited.
I stand with Christ at the top of the hill overlooking the beautiful grounds.
A wave to an old gent sitting at the grape arbor praying.
A walk among the saints; Saint Ignatius, Saint Francis Xavier, Saint Francis of Assisi.
An evening meal with friends then rest.

04/22/94 – A Refreshing Shower Begins Day 2

A refreshing shower then I begin to read the gospel according to Luke. As I read Chapter 5 verse 10, the words "Do not be afraid, from now on you will be catching men." causes chills to run over my body and a sense of purpose fills me and I begin to write in my journal. God's call is powerful yet frightening as it will change my whole life from this day forward. I must follow His call. I continue to read Luke 5 at the Call of Levi (verses 27 and 28) "He said to them, "Follow me," And leaving everything behind, he got up and followed Him." I once again felt the chill and goose bumps cover my flesh.

In Luke 6 Christ talks of love of your enemies and teaches us to give verse 30 reads, "Give to everyone who asks of you, and from the one who takes what is yours do not demand it back." I therefore must love Jack and give Jean to him freely and I must not demand her back. She will only return to me if her own free will chooses to return. I am being asked to give up all that is mine and to follow my God from now on. I cannot deny this call any longer.

I go out for a short walk and to pray at my grassy knoll for direction. As I lay there with God the image of Christ's face appears in the clouds. I see His pained face at the crucifixion, His deep saddened eyes bearing the pain of mankind's sins. I tell Him I will do whatever He directs me to do, I will follow Him to the ends of the earth. As His image drifts away, the image of Satan forms; pointed chin, hateful eyes, two prominent horns. I look upon his image and renounce him telling him I will fight against him with all my soul and that God's children will defeat him wherever he may appear. As I tell him to leave me his image distorts in anger and dissolves in God's winds. The image of Christ returns this time much larger than before with a look of peace upon His face. I feel He is smiling on me this morning with approval. I feel full of God's grace. God has once again overflowed my cup and let me feel His love into my very soul. I am at inner peace.

04/23/94 – Day 3 – A Day of Sharing

Breakfast is shared with friends. Vocational calls are discussed. I share my visions, Hobie shares one of his poems:

04/23/94 – Hobie Shares His Poetry

I ran from death, but death caught me
And asked me why I ran.
I ran from pain, but pain stopped me
And told me who I am.
I ran from God, but God held me
And begged me not to run.
"Let go of life and simply be,
My prodigal, my son."

54

Inner Work

04/24/94 – Sunday – Final Thoughts

I take a walk to be with God.
The birds are singing cheerfully.
The soft breeze and hum of bees soothe.
I sit with Mary on a hillside.
I pray and talk with God.
I pick an eleven-leaf clover.
A bubbling brook talks to the woods.
A woodpecker knocks at God's door.
The fresh air invigorates the soul.
I stop to speak to Joseph in the dale.
Joseph's lineage goes back to Seth.
Christ's human father was good.
All occurrences in the past mesh.
I smile at Mary in the Grotto,
There she stands in radiant white
The sun shines on her brightly.
My grassy knoll where visions lay.
A visitor greets me with "Good morning, Father"
I answered Good Morning naturally
My call is being confirmed everywhere.
Hobie has left a copy of his poems.
His writings touch my heart.
I gift him with my writings.
An invigorating bike ride around the grounds.

Inner Work

04/25/94 – I Blow up at Jean and Jack

Last night I blew up at Jean and Jack. They returned from their Spiritual Growth Retreat at 10 PM. I was upstairs while they let the dog out. About 10:30 Moxie's barking to be let back in was driving me up the wall so I went down to let him in. As I passed the front door, I saw Jean and Jack embracing in front of the house and kissing. I stood there for a minute or two then let Moxie in. I went out front then angry and inquired as to why Jack and Jean had to passionately kiss in front of the house with the porch lights on for everyone to see. Jean said he wasn't kissing her only hugging her and I got angry at her for lying to me. Why doesn't she just go and stop hurting me. It seems every time I come to grips with reality Jean beats me over the head again to inflict pain. What did I do to deserve this? I look out this evening at the full moon and it is beautiful. The screen causes the light radiating from the moon to form a perfect cross of light in the sky reaching from East to West and North to South. Venus shines brightly in the upper left quadrant of the cross. I feel good looking out at the cross in the sky. God seems to give me signs often to let me know He is here with me and that I should be more peaceful inside. I will pray again for His help through the pain. I know now that Jean will not return to me and I must move on with my life. Please God take care of Jean I do not wish her pain or harm. I watched The Wonder Years alone this evening. It was their daughter's wedding and I cried helplessly as I heard the vows being read. I only wish ours had remained sacred.

Inner Work

04/26/94 5:30 AM - Tears of Goodbye to Love (poem)

I lay here in bed, tears freely flowing.
These past months of loss have been hell.
I asked Jean for a hug early this morning.
As I held Jean close my heart did swell.
Mistakes of the past have poisoned her love.
I watch as my life's mate leaves for another.
My prayers for reunion seem unheard above.
Counselors and friends say, "Don't even bother."
No one on earth understands my commitment
To a woman who rejects my every attempt
To rekindle a love that God's angel sent
The eighteenth of May that bicentennial year.
I pulled Jean close to me early this morning.
I heard her gentle heart beating softly within.
A familiar sound from the past I will miss.
I don't want to let go and be lonely again.
I lay here in bed, tears freely flowing
Mourning the death of a heavenly union,
Praying for help as my heart is breaking.
God's love to you Jean, I'll miss you forever.
Please understand, I meant you no harm.
I don't wish you pain only life's happiness.
If life without me frees your child's spirit,
Then my holding on will only suppress
Your growth and cause pain I cannot permit.
My butterfly spreads her wings to the sky,
She flies for her freedom away from my heart.
I lay here alone with tears in my eyes,
My loneliness begins as now we must part.
Counselors and friends say "Trust in the Lord"
That's all I have left to fill in Jean's void.

Inner Work

05/01/94 - Breakfast at Bob Evans

Breakfast before church at Bob Evans. I was reviewing my typed journal and my waitress says, "Working so early on Sunday?" I replied "No, just reviewing a book I'm working on about men in midlife crisis." She started asking about how does one cope with a man in midlife who runs off with a woman younger than his daughter. We talked for a few moments and I told her to look after herself and not concentrate on her ex-husband and his girlfriend because she was OK. She thanked me as I left for church. She seemed relieved to know how to cope better with her pain. I feel God once again has put someone in my path to point the direction of my vocation out to me. I led this morning's adult Sunday school and the topic was "Companions Along the Way." It was a great session of inner work for all and it strengthened my belief in my desire to change my vocation in the near future.

05/02/94 - Driving in a Car (dream)

Driving in a car on a superhighway towards an island in the middle of a large river. I am being observed by people from both sides of a conflict. They seem to need to know my every move and my final destination. I cross the bridge to the island as the river rises to cover the road behind me, as I look back I realize that I am the last person to cross that bridge and my mission is critical and the information I am to receive on the island has to be delivered in person by me to a distant place. I pick up the information in a cave at the center of the island. Several foes are shot around the cave opening to let me escape. Their bodies fall into a deep chasm to the left of the opening. I am aware that the information I carry is not of this world and should not matter (in my opinion) to the opposing forces who are trying to stop my journey. I leave the cave with a partner to an airstrip and we get in a twin engine four seat aircraft and prepare to take off. The weather is extremely stormy, and visibility is poor, but we take off anyway. As we head across the river towards the mountains, we crash with neither opposing forces aware of where we crashed. I am the only survivor of the crash. A trucker stops on the road nearby and pulls me out of the wreckage and drives me to a nearby town. I meet two elderly women at the airport who must fly to their destination because of some urgent need there. It is their first flight and they are both afraid to fly. I purchase a seat near them and assure them that they will be OK. As we prepare to land the ladies become very panicky and afraid, I comfort them by talking to them and they thank me saying "You have a kind, soft and gentle voice that soothes when you speak, thank you for caring." We land safely, and I wake up.

Inner Work

05/16/94 - Jack Stayed at our House

Yesterday I returned from a week away and found out Jack had spent the week sleeping at our house. I feel as though I have been robbed. My sanctuary has been violated and I have been raped. Jean did not seem to understand my anger and pain at the results of here him visiting Jack to live in my house while was out of town. I feel they have given my children and their friends a very poor example of morals. I hurt so deeply inside. Jack not only has taken the woman I love from my life, but he has violated the sanctity of my home. I feel that I have nothing now, my home is not a comfortable place to be any longer. Dear God, when will this all end. I am being extremely patient waiting for your help but every where I turn more pain is found. I am not a rich man God, so I cannot afford the luxury of getting things done swiftly in today's costly world. Please help me get through this latest ordeal with some vestige of hope for the future.

05/17/94 - Another Fire Dream

Another fire dream, walking down a residential street when I hear fire sirens. Several fire trucks pass by and head towards a fire in a housing project across some railroad tracks. I rush to help other volunteers at the fire scene. We are stopped while a train goes by. I remember hearing the fire company alarms before the trucks appear and counting them saying "That's four alarms. There must be a huge fire nearby."

05/23/94 - Searching Deep in a Cave (dream)

Searching deep in a cave. I see creatures from mythology, minotaurs and cyclops, creatures with tortoise shells and winged creatures. This winged creature and this tortoise shelled creature have come to meet a challenge. I am a companion of the tortoise shelled creature who seems to be very knowledgeable of the upcoming challenge. They both approach the altar from opposite sides to prepare. Each looks into a mirror on their side of the altar to see what they will look like at the end of their journey and challenge. The tortoise shelled creature sees himself while the winged creature sees no reflection. The leader of the winged creatures says, "It is always like this, they both leave on their quest, but my beautiful winged child never returns." The winged creature preparing for the challenge vows to be successful and return to let others know what happens. I walk with my companions from the labyrinth and we journey to a majestic mountain where we find a large altar, taller than us all. We stand in front of the altar and a voice speaks to us, "Approach the altar and walk through and I will see you on the other side." We look at each other with confusion but proceed to walk to the altar one by one. The winged creature touches the altar and his hand disappears into the masonry. He recoils in fear. The tortoise shelled creature walks to the altar with me and says, "Let us pass through" and we both step through the altar beckoning to the winged creature as we enter. He follows us in. As we emerge on the other side, I feel full of life, the tortoise creature seems the same but the winged creature has shorn his wings and taken on human form completely. He looks exactly like me. We are all aware of the presence of God on this side of the great altar. The tortoise shelled creature knows he must return to the cave to guide the next journeyman to the altar. I now join hands with my transformed winged creature knowing we will not return to the cave altar as we now understand what happens each time the winged companion leaves with his human counterpart. As we stand there in God's light the tortoise leaves and our two bodies combine, and I feel whole and full of God's grace. As I wake up I feel anxious for my next challenge in life. My level of anxiety recently has been so high that I feel ready to jump out of my skin. I await God's guidance in life.

06/04/94 - Aunt Rita called

At dad's house, Aunt Rita called because mom's birthday would have been tomorrow. She asked me how everyone was. When she asked me how Jean was, I said, "Moving out!" she was shocked. I told her of my retreat experiences and my visions of late. She related to me things my mom constantly told her that I was not aware of. Mom constantly reminded Aunt Rita that deep inside Frankie is still very much a Catholic and deeply religious. Aunt Rita said maybe mom is working hard up there in heaven to pull me in the direction I should be going, if so the last year is more explainable but no less painful.

06/09/94 - "Cousins Tour 1993" T-shirt

I am going to Sherry Harbaugh's this evening to discuss Saint Timothy's dream workshop ideas then to Joan Appleton Jones' to fix her computer. Jean asks if it is OK for Jack to come by as she is watching the boys. I say OK, before I leave Jack shows up wearing the "Cousins Tour 1993" T-shirt from last summer. I feel pain deep in my heart as he proudly wears a shirt that says, "This is the weekend I stole Jean's heart from you." I say nothing and leave. Sherry and I talk of dream work and I see our friendship as a source of healing. I fix Joan's Windows software then we talk. Joan and I have been very close this last month. She listens to me and I to her. We are both searching for inner answers. She is an even greater source of healing. I am learning that my perception of myself in other's eyes has been wrong for a long time. Most people I have talked to have a much higher opinion of me than I had supposed. I feel better about myself.

Inner Work

I tell Jean about my pain yesterday at Jack's T-shirt and she says he did not mean to hurt me by wearing it he just wore it. Before I left for the Dream Retreat Jean told me she was moving the family room furniture while I am away and that she planned to take Tony with her and spend the weekend at Jack's. I leave for my retreat in great pain knowing that when I return the room in which we spent many days curled up in each in each other's arms and celebrated family Christmases will be empty. My heart has been emptied some more and pain has filled the emptiness. I arrive at Wernersville at 2 PM and go to my oak and my grassy knoll for reflection. I sit on a park bench for 3 hours and feel a great weight in my chest and deep loneliness in my heart. This weekend is going to be difficult. I show Sara (Jack's sister) and Rita around the grounds. Sara's presence may cause me some conflict, but I must look beyond that and concentrate on my retreat. We meet for two hours to prepare ourselves for our healing dream. I take a ritual bath to slowly cleanse myself in preparation for sleep, perchance to dream.

06/11/94 – Day 1 - Dream Retreat Begins

I awake at 7:15 hungry for breakfast. I slept a very sound sleep undisturbed by any inkling of a dream. After breakfast (Sara sat across from me) I went back to my room and lay on my bad and cried for an hour. I do so miss Jean and I realized that last night she slept a full night in another man's arms. I must look past this pain. I go out to my grassy knoll, it is overcast with a soft breeze blowing. I lay down as I have in the past, stretch out my arms and ask God to wash my sins away and a gentle rain begins to that lasts for about a minute. I thank God for cleansing me and pray for His guidance. I walk to the statue of Mary and the infant Jesus to pray and look over the valley below. I pick a strand of wheat and chew on it as I walk back to the Novitiate. As I approach the building Christ's image appears in the clouds to the right of the building and I thank Him for being there for me as I go through my pain. His image seems to be softly smiling at me as if to say "I am her for you son. I will hold your hand as you walk, and I will carry you if you falter. Your faith will be your strength." I feel better inside as I prepare for a short meeting with Bob.

61

Inner Work

I review my dreams of the past few months:

Fire dream	In a valley
Goddess Dream	She melts into me and caresses me
Climbing a tree	Embraced by the tree
Funeral dream	buried alive
Journey over mountains	Rain and mud below God above
Basement of new building	Child evaporates
Schooner	Going to a black hole
Car over river	Into a cave
Searching cave	Tortoise and winged transformation

Bob and I talk about past problems and I tell him I slept soundly. I feel this is going to be a weekend of rest rather than discovery. Bob says that might be good considering all my hard work over the past months. He suggests I don't concentrate on anything only enjoy the time here and get some much-deserved rest, basically to let my mind clear. I go back to my room and fall asleep. I awake at 12:15 and go to lunch. More sleep without dreams. I feel very relaxed. After lunch I return to my room to take a nap. It seems that this weekend I am to get a lot of sleep. Just as I think my weekend will be one of total relaxation all hell breaks loose internally, psyche bombards me with dreams and the process of internal healing begins.

At a Bar Gambling - Dream Retreat Dream #1

I dream that I am sitting at a bar gambling, playing tickets of chance. I seem to win often and the others around me are jealous. I open one ticket and it is a king (not a winning ticket). I start to discard it when I notice the edge is loose and realize that there is another chance hidden beneath. Beneath the king is a queen which is a winning ticket. I return to my room to rest (in my dream). I am just about to fall asleep when I notice a beautiful young woman (my goddess) in bed with me, she says, "I'm naked, I'm moist, make love to me!" I am startled as she was not there when I came into the room. She starts to take my clothes off. My shirt sleeves are difficult to pull over my hands. It seems almost impossible to get undressed. As I remove my clothes, she starts jumping around in the bed saying, "I'm 15 and I am going to be made a woman by this man." I think for a moment and say, "You're 15 and are too young to have sex with me." Somehow, I am convinced that it will be OK if we have sex. She helps me pull my socks off and seems very frustrated at how difficult it is to pull them off my feet. I go over to lock the door, so we are not disturbed, and she is looking out the window. "Your dog is outside with his towel and getting it dirty." she says. I tell her it's OK he plays with it all the time. We get in bed and she is clothed in a simple dress. I help her get undressed. I have difficulty with her bra, so she removes it. I slip her panties off and slip her dress over her head. I start to kiss her breasts and she says, "Don't hurt my boobies make love to me." I touch her moist vagina with my fingers and she pushes my hand into her saying, "Make me feel good, come into me, don't make the bed messy as I am afraid I did mine, make me a woman." As I start to make love to her, I recognize her voice as Phaedra's. I awake

Note: When I first noticed the woman in bed with me, I felt her vagina with my hand. It was hot and moist. My fingers easily slipped into her and she pressed her full breasts against my chest. As I undressed her later and started to kiss her breasts, they were small and not fully developed as a young teen's. Her vagina, while warm and moist, was smaller and my fingers did not fit easily into her. I feel the earlier body I touched was more mature to lure me into the experience. The person I made love to was definitely a young woman in her teens.

It is 3:30 and I must see Bob. He is talking with someone outside. I stop far enough away to keep from disturbing them. I pull up a chair in the passageway and look out at my mighty oak in the rain. Bob and I talk a short while. My dream is definitely to heal my inner wound. My wife is moving out this weekend while I am on retreat. Psyche gifted me with a nubile partner in my dreams to compensate for my loss.

Personal reflections: Nine months ago, on the first weekend of September my wife left for the beach inwardly saying she would not return emotionally to our marriage. At the beach she fell in love with another man and this weekend while I am here, she is moving into his house. This is the pain I am struggling with inside. This external painful situation has forced an extrovert to look inward for answers and God has helped me greatly. In the last several months I have had 8 dreams in which my feminine side has addressed me as a goddess, a child, a bride, a woman giving birth, a companion. But yesterday in the ninth month of pain the ninth dream came to me to heal me. She seduced me as a goddess then transformed into a 15 year old virgin excited that I was going to make her a woman. My healing dream of self-fulfillment of my masculine and feminine sides has compensated for the external pain by giving me great internal peace and satisfaction.

06/12/94 - Dream Retreat Day 2 03:00 AM
A Large Corporation (dream & analysis)

I am with 3 companions. We have come to a large corporation to visit an important person. The facility is securely guarded, and we have no passes. We set up a camp fire near the main building and are cooking food. A security guard asks us how we got in because the employees have noticed us and are afraid because they do not know who we are. I explain that one of the executives is expecting us and he will be out soon. My companions are going back and forth to our vehicle (outside the compound) to bring more equipment and food without being questioned. It seems as if we can pass through the security check area without being seen. Finally, the executive comes out to see us and picks up a plate to fill with food. He makes up an ample portion of all that is there and hands the plate to me and says, "Here eat, this food is for you." As I take the plate, I notice that it is only me and the executive, my 3 companions who were there as he approached seemed to have vanished into thin air. I start to eat the scrumptious meal and I wake up. I remember that one of my companions was a woman because she reprimanded one of the others for turning a dish of food upside down and he laughed because even with turning the bowl upside down the contents did not fall onto the ground but stayed in the bowl only to be removed by serving it with a spoon. I remember thinking how odd that nothing spilled as the contents were not sticky or real solid but more like a salad or cole slaw which would have easily been poured out.

NOTE: From the gate to the building was a curved access road going uphill. We were set up at the curve in the road near the crest of the hill.

04:00 AM - Laying in Bed Wide Awake

Laying in bed wide awake, tears flowing as I think of returning home to a partially empty home. I ask God what he wants of me as I am aware that something special is happening within me. As I ask the question the dream from my youth passes my mind. The elevator dream I was reminded of when Sherry related her elevator dream to me last Thursday evening. My dream reoccurred several times during my teen years, the time when I was seriously contemplating and preparing for the priesthood.

Inner Work

My Elevator Dream (dream & analysis)

There are two identical buildings like twin towers in a large hotel complex. Both towers have a glass elevator shaft facing into a common courtyard. As I get in one of the glass elevators to go to the top floor, I am aware that you can see everything through the glass in all directions. As we get to the top floor the elevator starts to go sideways and travels to the other tower. As we start to transverse from one tower to the other, I am afraid as the elevator floats from one to the other with no visible means of support. Once we begin to float though I am no longer afraid, and I enjoy the view from above. I also remember that if you stopped at a floor to go to your room it didn't matter what your room number was it was always directly in front of the elevator when it stopped. As I remembered my dream from my youth, I stepped out of one of the floors in my memory and noticed that I was collecting clothes for those in need. I only accepted clothes from those who could spare them and refused to take them from those who I felt could not spare them. I am reaching for some clothing being handed to me from a person on a tier above me and I notice the wall and the ground around me is covered with poison ivy which I am allergic to but I feel no fear as I am aware that I cannot be harmed by it as I am doing God's work. This seemed so real I had to write it down.

I return to sleep to dream once again.

I have two dreams with my teenage son Michael in them. They seem to happen in reverse order. In the first dream he is upset at his job that his timeslip does not reflect his overtime hours. I am standing with him as he confronts his supervisor who ignores him. I suggest he talk to the owner. It takes some prodding, but he goes to the owner who listens to him then we three go to confront the supervisor who does not seem to want to discuss the situation in front of me, but the owner makes him. He apologizes to Michael for his oversight and corrects the timeslip all the time glancing uncomfortably at me. I half wake up then fall back to sleep and dream again of Michael. This time he is applying for the job. His appointment is with a Mr. newton, who appears and is indeed Mr. Newton my favorite science teacher from high school. He is immediately impressed with Michael and hires him. Mike is introduced to his supervisor who is a couple of years older and obviously controlling but at the same time insecure in his position. He shows Mike around with Mr. Newton and I walking with them. he seems very uneasy that Mike has an easy time understanding the job being described to him. The supervisor again keeps glancing at me with a look of uneasiness sometimes even panic.

65

NOTES:

> 1) My son Michael as a teenager is the spitting image of me. His high school picture and mine could be put side by side and unless you noticed the age of the photos you could not tell the difference.
>
> 2) Mr. Newton was my very favorite science teacher in high school. I spent many extra hours after school working on projects with him.

07/02/94 - A Hillside Covered with People (dream)

I see a hillside covered with people. At the bottom of the hill the people I see are all women, twenty or thirty women and they are all perfect and naked. I seem to know that they are all virgins waiting for something special to happen. They are laying there as a great white wave caresses them. The wave was sperm and they all become pregnant at the same time and they all looked full of peace and love. There seems to be a Godly presence on the mountain. I am telling everyone to line up as in a choir, so I can lead them and teach them. The people on the hillside are asking me how to deal with pain, sorrow, anger and suffering. I tell them all to concentrate on their pain and bring it inward and hold it in for a moment then sing out their pain in praise to God. As they all do as I teach them an angelic chorus fills the air and the sound of the voices of the multitude is glorious and their pain is relieved. I notice they all sing the same words as happened in my past on a Mountainside in West Virginia. Everyone has felt deep inner healing and a closeness to God that they have never felt before. I tell them all to take what they have learned and pass it on to everyone whom they come in contact -with in hopes that if all learn to deal with pain, anger and suffering by offering it up to God in joyous song that the world will be healed of its sinfulness and the glory of God will be felt upon the earth.

I am going to miss Joan while she is out of town this weekend. She fills me with great joy and feelings of peace. I enjoy our conversations, our spirituality and our sexuality together. She has brought me out of the desert into a beautiful world of mutual understanding and respect. Our relationship is very special and important to me. I enjoy the sunshine that emanates from her smiles and laughter as it is given freely and with love to one so unworthy.

Inner Work

07/04/94 - Happy Birthday America!!

Today is a wonderful day Tony is here with me and Michael's friends are enjoying fireworks in the yard. Tony and I pick up Joan and go to watch the fireworks on City Island. We stop on a hillside in Camp Hill and sit on a blanket eating fruit and enjoying the fireworks display. It seems so natural to be here with Joan sitting on a blanket, I really enjoy her presence. We go back to the house and sit out back watching the kids set off fireworks. The boys all go swimming and we laugh at their antics. It is a beautiful night and I feel a closeness that I have not felt for a long time and it feels good.

07/08/94 - To Wernersville with Joan.

The ride to Wernersville with Joan is delightful. She and I communicate so well with each other, neither of us confine the other with boundaries or insurmountable expectations. We are going for a silent overnight spiritual retreat. We arrive at the Jesuit Center and as usual the serenity of the entrance road caresses me and holds me in its bosom. We check in to get our room assignments and then I walk with Joan around the grounds to share with her the realm of my dreams. I show her my oak tree, grassy knoll, Mary's grotto (my bride in radiant white), Joseph's circle (Seth's ancestor), the path past a small creek. We pick blackberries and raspberries and share God's gift of life and love. After we bring our bags into our rooms, I seek out Father Aschenbrenner for brochures that Joan needs about the Center. After meeting with Father Aschenbrenner we go out again to see more of the grounds, the Cloister walk, the statuary, the arbor. We stop by the swimming pool and meet Toshi there. He is in his last week of training before returning to Hiroshima. We go to dinner together and sit with Toshi and Jeff (a retreatant who enjoys the talking meal as a break from his silence.) Conversation at dinner is gentle as Joan and Jeff talk of Lock Haven, PA and their mutual contact with a Lutheran pastor. Joan sparkles as she talks of a jazz minister, she heard there last weekend. Dinner is done, and silence begins. We part company and go our separate ways to quietly commune with God and ourselves. I relax in my room and start to read "Original Blessing" by Matthew Fox. It is a book sent to jean by Andrea Thomas her friend in Ohio. The book is captivating but sleep quickly overwhelms me and I rest.

Inner Work

07/09/94 – Early Shower then Visit My Grassy Knoll

An early shower and a visit to my grassy knoll to pray. I walk to the statue of Mary with the infant Jesus and watch the sunrise. It is so beautiful here, the sun cresting behind the clouds sending rays of light through the sky. God once again welcomes His creation to a new day. Breakfast is in silence, Joan sits at a different table as we share smiles of Good Morning without sound. I am glad she wanted to come here and share my world of peace, sanctity and spirituality. We have become very close these last six weeks and I know that I can trust her with my heart. After breakfast I take my book outside to read. Joan is taking a bike ride, I hold the door for her and she rides off toward the cemetery. I sit and read occasionally looking up at my mighty oak. I see Joan racing down the hill on the bike, she throws her head back and coasts with the breeze pushing her hair back. She is so full of life and love I know our friendship will be long lasting and fulfilling. I notice our level of connectivity is very deep and is of great comfort to me in this time of rebirth. I thank God for allowing us to "bump into each other." Joan is truly one of God's gifts in my life. As I read "Original Blessing" I become more aware of my recent growth in spirituality and my contact with my feminine side. The many references to Julian of Norwich remind me of my Comic Book dream in which my feminine gave birth to Julian and the connection pulls me deeper into the book. Creation-Centered Spirituality is the future.

07/23/94 - A Carnival Like Atmosphere (dream)

A strange dream, a carnival like atmosphere, different competitive games going on; racing, boxing (if you can call either event observed by those names). the racing is horse racing where the fans are right at the edge of the track and they taunt and distract the riders and horses as they pass. The fans derive great pleasure from this distraction. Several times a horse and rider fall, in one instance the rider is trammeled to death by the following mass of horses. The next horse who falls the rider seems attached to the saddle and cannot get loose. There is panic in his face as he hears the others coming. A group of fans rush onto the track to try to drag horse and rider out of the way. The succeed in getting the horse to stand, the rider is facing backwards as the horse continues the race. The next scene is an arena where boxing matches are being held. A match just ended with one contestant dead. The next pair was a tall man, well-built and a short, out of proportion man. He looked like a dwarf, small childlike body with oversized adult head. The dwarf is wobbling back and forth like a weeble doll the kids use to have, his head bobbing out of balance back and forth. The tall man is yelling "Make him stop that, I cannot fight him while he is doing that." The contestants are told to leave the arena as the announcer announces the final match. This is a similar match up only the dwarf has both hands heavily bandaged. They are led to the center of the ring where they are asked to compete in a glass bell which gives them little room to move. The taller man keeps taunting the dwarf, "Hit me first so I can hit you back. I cannot hit you first you are smaller than I am." The dwarf holds both hands together and swings his whole body in circular motion and swings at the tall man but misses him and his hands hit and shatter the glass bell. The dwarf says, "Let's stop this circus. I am a representative of the owner and she wishes to stop all the competition. There have already been three deaths and we do not need a fourth." They leave the ring and exit by way of a staircase against the wall. The wall is curved as the room is circular and the stairs are spiral going up. One cannot see the top of the spiral stairs only notices images on the wall as they go up. The images are a chronology of the carnival. The images change according to whomever is climbing the staircase. It seems that the images reflect the climber's life in the carnival shifting scenes as one goes up reflecting their life. If one stood still on the staircase and looked up and down the scenes on the wall one could observe their own life past, present and future. I awake as the audience is pleased that the carnival is stopped. I notice that I am half way up the staircase when I wake up and had just looked up at the images of the future. I had not had time to focus on the images, but I know they seemed different than those depicting the past. The image of the present was of course the carnival and the total chaos and confusion present there just prior to the decision to stop the circus and stop the killing.

Inner Work

07/24/94 - Sailing on a Large Lake or Sea (dream)

Sailing on a large lake or sea, I am on the bow controlling the sail as we (four-man crew) move swiftly in the gentle breeze. We head towards a dam or spillway on the far side of the lake. As we approach the shallow water, I am alone at the center of the boat lifting the centerboard to prevent it from scraping bottom. At the dam I lower the sail, lift the centerboard out and put both in the hull and secure them to the boat. I push the boat through a spillway to send it to the water below as I walk down the cliffs on the right to get down to the river below. The sailboat is drifting towards a shallow eddy on the far side of a bend in the river. I walk along the shore to go pick up my sailboat. I notice that in one area I must wade in the river (water comes up to my waist) to reach my destination. At the far side of the bend I gather in my sailboat and rest calmly on the shore enjoying the beauty of the wilderness around me. I wake up. The funny thing about this dream is that the river area and spillway were very familiar to me, I have either actually been in that place several times before or I had dreamed the exact same journey several times in my youth.

07/29/94 - Driving a Car Fast Through Town (dream)

Unusual dream. Driving a car fast through town, passenger and I must make a train at station across town. Passenger is escorting me to an interview for a job as Director of Personal Computer Operations. We arrive at the train station 10 minutes late for the train, but a Redcap says don't worry the train is running late and it is still in the station. We run to the platform just as the train starts to move. We jump onto the train, there is no top on the cars almost like cars of a roller coaster. The seats are narrow, and we have difficulty squeezing into them, but we manage to get on board as the train leaves. We are in the last car of the train, no roof above us but I notice a large wasp or hornet's nest above me (suspended in space basically). I hit at the nest to make the wasps or hornets leave it. The passengers around me are afraid they will get stung by the insects, but I calm them by saying, "Don't worry they will not sting you the train is moving swiftly, and they will be blown away by the wind. The insects do come out of the nest and circle us they land on my arms but do not sting me. They seem peaceful and unwilling to harm me or anyone on the train. I shoo them away and the train continues on as I wake up.

70

Inner Work

10/02/94 - Course in Miracles Class

Abigail gave a touching account of her experience in Germany where she communicated with a Russian soldier who said, "We are people, we are only people." After her description of her encounter she asked if everyone was O.K., I obviously was not. The experience brought back an episode I had 32 years ago as a teenager in Japan. I was visiting Hiroshima, as I walked down the street where you could see the coal black shadows of people instantaneously obliterated by the atomic bomb I experienced a feeling of awareness of the presence of many people calling to me. As I listened to the story about the Russian soldier that sensation returned, and I was back in Hiroshima listening to the cries of "We are people, we are only people." emanating from the shadows around me. I once again felt the presence of multitudes in pain not understanding their rapid departure from this earth. I then recollected my "Musings on Death" I wrote last week, and the images of Hiroshima became clearer. The atomic explosion evaporated thousands of people in a blinding flash of intense white light, all those souls being released at once. The most vivid image I remember is the shadow of a woman bending over her young child to shield the child from danger. This shadow was burnt into the white mortar wall next to the road on the crest of a small knoll. If I turned around with the shadows to my back, I was looking directly at the blackened skeleton of the only building left standing after the blast "GROUND ZERO". As I closed my eyes, I felt at one with the child whose shadow was behind me. I could see the mushroom shaped cloud, the great flash of light, barely hear the wailing of the air raid sirens because the cries of the people were too loud but I never heard the explosion from the bomb because the sound passed by after I was evaporated by the heat. During that moment of reflection, I could fell the great rush of cosmic wind that passed over this city that August day 49 years ago. I was there at the moment of release. After class Joan and I talked on the way home and it finally occurred to me why I have always had a great affinity for the Japanese people, enjoyed learning their culture and visited their land four times in my lifetime. Hiroshima was bombed in August of 1945 and I was born in December of 1945 my soul was either present at Hiroshima or in intimate contact with the soul of that young child whose mother's body could not protect him from the ultimate destruction that was failing from above. I was gifted with the knowledge of their experience at birth. I know I have been put here with a special purpose to fulfill, that being to spread the truth to people about the need for love to be the means for all communication. I know that hate and anger and pain can be dealt with by bringing it inward immediately, holding it in for a moment to become one with it then letting your soul channel it through your heart to transform it into love and gentleness and soothing grace to bring peace to yourself and those around you.

1995 DREAMWORK PROSE and POETRY

Overview of 1995

The year 1995 was to be a year of increased growth and revelation. My vision of God's forgiveness and how I handle pain and anger struck me like a bolt of lightning. For the first time, I recognized my wholeness and the many gifts God gave me throughout life.

My dreams recorded during 1995 are incomplete due to a file I lost while using my laptop computer as a recording media. I vowed from that point on to write all dream occurrences on paper before putting them into my computer.

The first half of 1995 I began to better understand my ability to deal with pain and anger. The Course in Miracles became even more important as a tool for self-healing and growth.

My dream of a quest with an angelic companion sets the stage for Dream Retreat #2 where I, through my dreams, start the restructuring of my life. Several of my dreams were only short snippets but nonetheless to the point, I was to move forward from that retreat and deal with the external life using the inner strength I had gained.

The second half of 1995 is missing unfortunately, but I know my sessions with Bob and the dreams we analyzed continued to enhance my growth.

Inner Work

03/12/95 – Tapestry of Illusion
We are each but a single thread in a tapestry of illusion woven across time by ego.
Frank J. Costanza

03/26/95 - A Course in Miracles
A note about the Tapestry and the Weaver

Tonight, in the Course in Miracles a revelation occurs. I now know how I handle pain and anger so well. I no longer will say that I do not know how I do it. I will explain it to anyone who cares to listen and let them try to comprehend. I used to say my gift was to be able to take anger, hurt and pain inward and transform it into song of praise to God but that is not entirely correct. My gift is to be able to take the anger, hurt or pain of the world of illusion inward and give it back to the author, my higher Self, and reject that part in the drama of life. I don't need to play the angry, hurt or painful role if I do not choose to live it. God's gift back to me is the expression of Joy in song that emanates from my lips and through my very soul. This is my blessing and gift from God.

04/14/95 - Walking with a Friend (dream)

My quote about the Tapestry of Illusion (03/12/95) came to me during the Course in Miracles session that night but tonight it came clear to me through my dreams. I dreamed I was walking with a friend to someone's house, as we approached the house an ice cream vendor passed on the next street. My companion ran to buy something for me from the vendor. She returned with a pair of wax teeth like the kind I remember from my childhood. I put them in my mouth as I approached the door to be funny and to see if the people inside would recognize me. Of course, I was recognized because the house I was entering was not of the world of illusion and all persons there were aware of themselves as described in my quote. "We are each but a single thread in a tapestry of illusion woven across time by ego." The scene immediately changes, and we were all in a large arena setting up a circus in which we were all entertainers. I woke up realizing that this whole world of illusion is like a circus in which ego moves us around from act to act and We can choose if we wish to play or not.

Our upper Self sets the stage, writes the play, directs the scene then hands the script to each of us in the world of illusion. We each in turn give that part over to ego who weaves the tapestry we see and feel and live. If we pull out our thread the tapestry unravels and the design changes as we are woven into the next tapestry only to unravel again

73

as we move on. Each time the tapestry unravels we learn and we also notice that each thread in the tapestry, each person in our tapestry, is an entity of its own with its own identity, beauty and author. I now know that I can unravel each tapestry and watch the weaver re-weave a new tapestry and enjoy the fruits of his labor. I await the beauty I know is coming nearer every day with great inner peace.

04/15/95 - Awareness Comes

I can now look back over my life and see the gifts God gave me from the very beginning. I am only now fully realizing the powers within that I can accept or reject. Last year I felt a great void when my marriage fell apart, but when I finally realized that I was complete in myself and did not need anyone in my life to fulfill it (to quote myself; "I do not need a woman in my life anymore and will never love one again!"), Joan came into my life. Our love for each other is strengthened by our knowledge that we are each complete as we are and that we do not need each other to be complete. We complement each other wonderfully.

05/08/95 - On A Quest with An Angelic Companion (dream)

I awake, it is 5 AM and I must write down my dream. On a quest, I am to journey through a beautiful forest to a lake in a lush verdant valley. The way is known if one doesn't try to think of how to go, but as one comes to each crossroads or fork in the road one closes their eyes and God shows the proper choice. I have a companion, a beautiful woman, or at least she seems to be a human woman. The journey is peaceful and the beauty around me is intense. We reach the valley of the lake and there are others there swimming in the lake. We are all nude swimming in the lake when I notice an opening in the side of the mountain where the source of the lake seems to be. We all enter the cavern via the water. It is a beautiful cavern and my companion, and I make love in the water. It is very fulfilling, and I realize my companion is not human but angelic in nature. The others notice this and warn me of an evil presence in the cavern that tries to destroy the angelic ones in front of their companions. I then notice another person there who is with my angelic companion and all of a sudden, he produces a gun and is going to kill her. I overcome him somehow and take his weapon from him. It is not like any gun I have even seen. It doesn't shoot bullets but if you shoot someone with it their spirit seems to wane, and they become very respondent to your commands. I use the gun to make him come with me as I must turn him over to the authorities to be placed in prison. He is taken away by the guards and I talk with one of the guards who says, "Thank you for returning him. He escaped this morning." As we were talking, my prisoner asked the other guards for a moment to stop at the other gate to look out at the beautiful scenery. They allow him to and he disappears into the forest. I mention this to the guard I was talking to and he said, "This happens all the time, the cycle begins over until the journeyer learns the meaning of the way he just traveled." I then explain to the guard my interpretation of the journey I just completed; "The journey I just traveled is my final journey of acceptance of God as my only true source of inner strength and my female companion is a guardian angel who helped me find the way each time I closed my eyes and asked inwardly for direction in life. The beautiful valley and crystal-clear lake were my glimpse of Paradise or Eden given to me as a reward for letting God show me the way. The cave was the source of all good and evil in my life. The evil person was the dark side of my free will, that tries to destroy our connection with the angels around us. The capture of this evil person was my inner victory over that side of me which pulls me from my God. The return of him to this prison was my releasing the power he had over me to God's guardian angels. As I related this revelation, the evil one reappeared at the other gate and was immediately recaptured by the guards and taken into the prison to be reformed and cleansed of all evil by God's grace. The guard smiled at me and my heavenly companion reappeared beside me and said, "We have made this same journey together many times and I am pleased that you have finally taken the time to understand its meaning. Others at the lake will continue this cycle until each one of them finally understands and accepts God as their way in life. I will always be with you wherever you journey."

Inner Work

06/16/95 – Opening session

We review the Asclepian method of incubating a dream and Bob tries something new this year. We each are asked to draw or paint a sketch of our dream goal for the weekend. I start by painting a large oak tree on a grassy knoll with a rainbow arching above rifling the upper two thirds of the paper. While brushing the finishing touches on the rainbow I feel the urge to draw on the lower third of the page three object on fire; the first object was a bottle of booze, the second a gambling ticket of chance and the third was a wad of dollar bills flying away. All three objects were engulfed in flames beautiful red, yellow and orange flames licking the green grass above them. I initial and date the lower right corner of the painting then add one finishing touch to the tree a burnt umber cross in the center of tree the directly above the burning debris of change below. My object for the retreat is to address new changes I want to begin within me to freshen my life and my future.

06/17/95 – 04:43 AM – Two dreams
Short snippet of a dream:

At home waiting for Jean to return Tony. Everyone is waiting for her arrival, roomful of people including Jack. Phone call to Jack's house to see if Jean has left yet. As the phone starts ringing Jean comes racing around the corner in her car. I hang up the phone and the dream is over.

Second dream:

Watching a new roof being put on a building across the way. The building is surrounded by large trees full of birds, very noisy birds flying around the roof in and out of holes in the roof. The workers don't seem to mind the birds and the birds don't seem to be disturbed by the workers hammering and sawing and stapling. The scene shifts, and I am on the roof observing the work being done. Bob Stoudt is there working on an overhang (Mansard style roof). I help to lay shingle on the last area to finish, it is an area to the lower left of where I am standing talking with the workers. They are relating a story of a spirit child named Tim who tries to stop or impede the progress of repairing the roof He pushes me in the back to try to make me lose my balance and fall off, but I don't. The way down from the roof is a spiral ramp or driveway. As I go down the ramp to the tunnel at the bottom Char and Jean are there. I relate the story of Tim and my experience to them and they just shrug it off. I go back up on the roof to look at the work. It is well done and complete. I am alone up here except for the feeling of the spirit's presence and all those noisy birds singing in the trees surrounding the building.

As I recall my dream, I remember that the spirit child Tim's antics of pushing and shoving people from behind was not to harm or throw them off the roof but the term mischievous kept coming to mind concerning him. As I lay here contemplating my dream the sky outside is slowly lighting with the first light of dawn and early birds are chirping happily outside.

06/17/95 – 09:30 – 10:00 AM – Session with Bob Stoudt

I show Bob my painting and express my goals for the weekend and my future; a new beginning and cleansing of my inner sell I relate both my dreams to Bob and I decided that rather than discuss the painting I would like to review my second dream. Bob asks me to relate various aspects of the dream as follows:

Describe the building: The building is old and the roof needs repair badly.

Mischievous child: Tim is 9 or 10 years of age and enjoys prodding people to distract them from their assigned tasks.

Trees and birds: The trees surround the building (a grove of large oaks) and are filled with beautiful songbirds singing away, flitting in and out of the boughs and the eaves of the root

The ramp down: A concrete spiral, maybe a driveway to the roof twisting down to the left into a tunnel below the building very steep at the top. Steep enough for one to be cautious not to slip when walking down it.

Bob and I analyze the dreams meaning. Bob asks me to describe the building as if I am the building:

I am an old building old enough to have watched the grove of trees around me grow from saplings to large full trees. My roof needs repair badly to protect the insides of the building. I feel great hearing the workers above fixing my hole ridden roof and the birds around generate music to my ears as I am repaired. They net in my eaves and bring forth new life each spring. I am in the middle of my useful life and the

77

repairs are needed to make me whole once again.

Bob asks about the mischievous child Tim:

Tim is a mischievous youth of about 9 or 10 years of age. He does not mean to harm the workers or myself only to slow down their process. I have known several Tims in my life;

Tim Gorka - President of Hycor the company the asset purchased my company (Productivity Center Inc.) and employed me as his company's Vice President until it fell into bankruptcy. Tim was meticulous to a fault, very controlling of his workers, with a good heart and generous. He was not the Tim of my dream.

Tim Salerno - Jean's nephew: youthful, quiet, maybe mischievous but I didn't know him well enough to relate him to the Tim in my dream.

Tim Carvey - my cousin: 9 to 10 years younger than me, one of 14 children of my Aunt Ginny and Uncle Eddie from Hydeville, Vermont (where I was born). Timmy was definitely the mischievous child of the family, always tagging along with Mickey, Bobby and I and being in the way when we were going to do something as a group. I think he most relates to the child in my dream.

Bob asks about me at 9 or 10 and also me 9 or 10 years ago:

Frankie at 9 or 10 is living in Virginia, attending Occoquan Elementary School, active in little league (pitcher and center fielder, pitched 32 games - 16 shutouts - batted well - place hit for singles and doubles) active Cub Scout, loved camping and the mountains (Shenandoah nearby). I had a girlfriend there (Nancy Ebert) she was older than me and 6 to 8 inches taller than me, so I would jump into her arms for a hug and kiss at the school playground or the bus stop. My best friend was Michael Jankowski who had polio, so his one leg was slightly deformed, but he was a friend you could always count on when you needed him. His father (Sergeant Jankowski U.S.M.C.) taught us how to fish and shoot a shotgun when we were 10. My dad would go on scout trips with us and mom was our Cub Scout den leader. Scouts were great fun. My baseball talents netted me a Baseball Scholarship to DeMatha Catholic High School, but my grades forced me to choose between academics and sports, academics won out, so I left DeMatha and went to public schools.

Frank 9 or 10 years ago (1985 - 1986) was a Systems Design Engineer at IBM Poughkeepsie (second time to Poughkeepsie previous stint I was a Design Technician). Between the assignments at

78

Inner Work

Poughkeepsie Jean and I were in Manassas where I was responsible for moving a component processing line from Burlington, Vermont to Manassas. We were on a one-year temporary assignment in Vermont that lasted only six weeks as Jean was scared by a snake in the back yard of a beautiful house we were renting in Underhill in the mountains (15 acres of land, trout stream, beaver dam at the bottom, ski area (Stowe) 30 minutes away). I had just recently been promoted from a non-exempt position to an exempt (professional) position in Manassas. My career was in transition. In 1985 1 was sent on a 12-day display tour of optical technology in Japan (Kobe, Osaka, Tokyo) all the top development labs that Japan had to offer. My task was to assess the technology and report back to the Vice President where the future of laser technology seemed to be heading. NOTE: I graduated from High School in 1963 from Misawa Dependents High School, Misawa AFB, Misawa, Japan. My senior class trip was a week in Tokyo with side trips to Kobe, Osaka, Mount Fuji and Hiroshima. My life is a continuing spiral around Japan, Vermont, Virginia, Maryland and New York.

Japan:
   1962–63 Misawa, Tokyo, Hiroshima – High School student
   1965–66 Atsugi, Hiroshima – United States Marine Corps
   1985   Kobe, Osaka, Tokyo – IBM Design Engineer

Vermont:
   1945–46 Born in Rutland lived in Hydeville at grandparents
   1982   IBM Burlington Senior Associate Programmer

Virginia:
   1951–58 Triangle and Occoquan – Elementary schools
   1982–83 Manassas – IBM Tech., Programmer, Engineer

Maryland:
   1959–62 Riverdale –Junior and Senior High School
   1967–76 Bethesda, Greenbelt – College, IBM   (Manned Space Flight)
   1982   Gaithersburg IBM Senior Lab Specialist (FSD)

New York:
   1977–82 Poughkeepsie   IBM Development Engineering (Technician)
   1983–88 Hyde Park - IBM Design Engineering (Design Engineer)

Bob observes from my comments that the house is middle aged and in need of repair as I am in the middle of my life and undergoing great change and transition also. Bob asks about me to describe what a roof means to me and how it relates to the inner me:

The roof is a protective device that prevents the insides from being damaged by the external elements, rain, wind, snow, etc. The roof is my mind the control area of my body. The need of repair is obvious if I look at my present state of transition. I am about to enter a new marriage and my house needs to be put in order, both 53 Honeysuckle and Frank. I need to focus more on repairs that are needed to move forward in life. The mischievous child is that inner child that distracts us from our tasks. Bob suggests that the child is trying to pull me away from the needed inner work (cleansing myself of the problems in my painting). While Bob talks, I feel heavy and tears fill my eyes for I know the child does not wish to harm me or stop my work. A realization surfaces: maybe just maybe the mischievous child's purpose is to slow down my inner process rather than impede it. He wants me to slow down rather than do as I always have and rush through the process of cleansing. I feel a deep hunger inside for healing and cleansing so that Joan and I might enter our new life with peace. I am reminded that the tasks of repairing 53 Honeysuckle and Frank are not something to be accomplished overnight but will take time and concerted effort to effect permanent growth.

06/17/95 – 16:45 – *Things Come into Perspective*

As I lay resting this afternoon thoughts of my dream and the session with Bob race through my mind. I nap but don't dream. I am totally exhausted today. My eyes are still heavy.
Two major things hit me:
First - There is another Tim in my life today that is very much a part of my life and who I am today, Saint Timothy Evangelical Lutheran Church or as we affectionately call it Saint Tim's.
Second - While watching this flood of thoughts race through my mind the initials that comprise the name TIM become apparent to stand for four phrases comprising of three words:

<u>Time Is</u> Meaningless
Today I Matriculate
<u>This Is</u> Miraculous
Timothy <u>Is Me</u>

I am a child of today, a pioneer in life
God's love flows over me every moment
I am full of life and growing constantly
I do not need the rest of the world to understand me
I am myself and I am pleased with who I am
My roof has been repaired now I must clean up the inner me
I go forth from here stronger than I entered here
The inner tasks never end they just transmogrify the outer me

Inner Work

06/18/95 – 00:45 AM – Confirmation Age Children at a Theater (dream)

With confirmation age children at a theater. They are going to sing on stage. We hear the piano being played I ask isn't that so-and-so then we see the piano. It seems to be a competition and the child playing the piano is on stage with his parents watching him play. The children and I are looking for our seats. We go into the vestibule and there are many of my confirmands there and they all appear slightly intoxicated holding drinks. Jamie says, "Here's Mr. Costanza let him by." I pass them to a table where the drinks are made. It is a large table full of all different bottle of booze. I pick up a drink and again start to follow a couple of the children into the auditorium to be sedated. It's like playing follow the leader up and down the aisles through rows of seats. The sections don't all seem to face the same way as if purposely confusing. I finally say enough of this game and throw my drink out and sit down to watch the others on stage. Everyone is happy and the music and singing on stage if beautiful. I awaken and must go to the bathroom.

06/18/95 – 02:30 AM – A Large Amphitheater (dream)

At the front of a stage in a large amphitheater full of children and their parents. There is a short partition like the orchestra pit in most theaters in the front to prevent the people from seeing those preparing to come on stage. I am watching what seems to be a competition of different kinds of acts. The show is to raise money for a charitable function. A friend of mine is on stage doing stand-up comedy. The emcee asks for a competitor to come up as no one has challenged this act. My friend sees me and tries to cajole me into performing in the competition against him. I am reluctant to go on stage, so they continue with other acts. Finally, my friend has convinced me to perform. I am introduced as the other comedy competitor. My act is introduced as Rhymes and Songlets from the past. I ask the adults to remember back to when their parents and relatives told them jokes and short poems to make them laugh then I started out with, "The other day upon the stairs I met a man who wasn't there. He Wasn't there again today. I wish to heck he'd go away." They all laughed remembering their youth and their children looked puzzled much as we did as youth the first time we heard that little ditty. I then sang "Marzy doats an dozy doats and little lamzy divy, a kidlil edvy too wouldn't you." fast so that the sentence was confusing to the children's ears and made no sense. Again, a puzzled look I said, "We'll return to that later and I started into, "Way in the morning in the

81

middle of the night. Two dead brothers got up to fight. Back to back they faced each other, drew their swords and shot each other. A deaf policeman heard the noise and came to arrest the two dead boys. If you don't believe this tale I tell ask the blind man he saw it all." The impossibility of each sentence made the children laugh and I beamed. I the repeated "Mares eat oats" fully as it was originally sung. The previous lines "Marzy doats an dozy doats and little lamzy divy, a kid 'Il edivy too wouldn't you." fast then very slow and determined, "If these words sound queer and funny to your ears, a little bit jumbled and jivey sing, "Mares eat oats and does eat oats and little lambs eat ivy. A kid'll eat ivy too wouldn't you." I brought one of the children up to do some of the senseless jokes my uncles used to do. Such as sit the child on a chair, ask him to concentrate on everything I do and say then with my one hand on his shoulder take my pointer finger of my other hand and bring it very chose to but not touch his nose. I then asked him, "Am I touching you as I circled my finger in front of his nose." He answered, "No." Then I started tapping him on the shoulder with the fingers of my other hand which was on his shoulder all the time. All the audience laughed, and my friend came up on stage and we went on doing jokes together and all had a great time.

06/18/95 – 06:00 AM – A Very Sexually Explicit Dream

I awaken in the middle of a very sexually explicit dream in which my partner and I are exploring all the different possible positions one can utilize for sexual intercourse. I never reached a climax only tried multiple positions to see how they felt to both of us. I awaken very aroused.

06/18/95 – 09:55 AM – A Short Nap Dreaming (dream)

I arise from a short nap dreaming. I seem to be very exhausted this whole weekend. My eyes constantly heavy, my chest heavy and a feeling of constant pressure on my bladder. I juke in my napping state and my legs pull up in a position of a woman on a delivery table. I rest my hands on the top of my head and slowly move my fingers over my head; the forehead my eyes and ears my nose my lips my throat. I start at the top of my chest and feel my body as pressure from above pushes downward toward my stomach. I slide my hand over my body caressing my abdomen as I fell a push outward. I grab my knees and pull my legs toward my chest. My body vibrates and my legs tingle as I feel pressure in my genitals. My legs spread a gap as I feel as though I am delivering a child. I feel lightened in both head and heart as I relax laying prostrate on my bed, a smile comes over my whole person and my thirst seems great. I feel whole and full of life. God has blessed me this weekend as he seems to do so often in my life. But this experience I have never felt before and the pleasure from deep within is undefinable.

06/18/95 – 10:30 AM – My final session with Bob.

We review my weekend and the dreams I recorded since our last session. My last dream of birth was the culmination of a powerful weekend of dream work and inner repair. Bob congratulates me on my retreat and the progress I underwent. I must now go forward and put into action in my outer life what my inner self has made me aware of concerning myself Psyche is telling me to go more slowly with myself I must listen to psyche as she knows me best.

1996 DREAMWORK PROSE and POETRY

Overview of 1996

The first quarter of 1996 seemed like a blur in time. My dreamwork had been set aside and life had been hectic at best. In ignoring my inner work, I noticed that the days were more filled with chaos and stress. I decided to therefore return to the regimen of the last couple of years and become reacquainted with the inner me, the more attune with the universe me.

Easter week of 1996 began my latest quest, internally, for explanation of my vocational "call". My dreams awakened my friend Psyche that I needed to find resolution to my questions. I began to feel the pull to open my arms wider and to help more people with their struggles.

The death of Joe Smith at the age of 38 inspired me to use my "Musings on Death" poem on a greeting card for expression of sympathy. It was to become my "Hallmark" of care and concern, touching the hearts of many who suffered loss of loved ones. My vocational "call" was starting to be fulfilled.

Although I did not have a great volume of dreams as in previous years, the dreams I did have were very developmental and gave me guidance when I needed it to move on in life. Psyche, I learned, is a relentless teacher and does not give up on me.

I open the chapter of written conversation with the inner self with a poem written as an apology to the one most important in my life and my guide to self-discovery, God.

Inner Work

An Apology to God

I write my apologies on the wind
    To the one above who never sinned
He leads me on with fire within
    To preach His word and share again
The inner work we each must do
    To find the drive to start anew
Looking inward for forces true
    To accomplish all God asks us to
To change the lives and ways of all
    To answer God's unwavering call
To spread the word and prove appall
    At mankind's invention of a fall
Since time began on this fair earth
    Humankind has questioned its own true worth
I profess we must discard this dearth
    Life with God within is one of mirth
A life so whole and full of grace
    That one can bear the darkest place
The worst life offers we can face
    When God's love within sets the pace
Forgiveness is a virtue found
    Love and care shall then abound
God's grace always will astound
    As ever onward we will bound
Moving toward that final day
    When all will come to see God's way
To join together and prayerfully say
    With God in heaven we are one today

Inner Work

04/04/96 (Maundy Thursday AM) - In a Conference Hall (dream)

In a conference hall in a large hotel. The room is a tiered amphitheater-like conference hall. The people are sitting in groups of two or three in very plush settees with short tables in front of them for their notes. I am asked by Paul Allair (Xerox Executive) to speak to the gathered group of marketing personnel. I start by talking of my time in research and development in the IBM labs. I tell of "prospecting" with ideas for new products. In the lab one would come up with ideas for new designs and scratch them down on paper and, with a little testing and rewiring, come up with a potential product. The prototype is then shown to marketing personnel and management to see if the idea will fly. I compare that background to what the marketing reps do when digging for leads. They scratch the surface prospecting and when a glimmer of gold appears, they pursue it more vigorously until they are rewarded with success. The audience seems to understand what I am telling them, and I return to my seat in one of the middle rows. Another person comes forward to lead the group in a song. He is pretty bad and cannot get the rhythm right or motivate the people. I am asked once again to come forward and lead. This time I begin to sing hymns of praise to God and all slowly join in until the room is full of glorious sounds of voices singing to God, thanking him for his love and blessings.

04/05/96 (Good Friday) - I Dreamt Again Last Night

I dreamt again last night, and I know the dream was short but significant. I cannot remember it now, but I can feel it pulling me inward again. I have not been faithful to my journalizing of dreams this past several months and it is time that I started writing again. This powerfully felt but not remembered dream seems to be pushing me onward. God does not seem to want to leave me alone. I am being called to lead in several places at once: At home with both the younger children and with the older more confused teen/young adult crowd that seems to have no direction in life; At work with helping new PC users become comfortable with their computers; At Saint Timothy's as Mutual Ministry co-chairperson, Stewardship committee person, choir member, council member and youth class facilitator; And outside of Saint Timothy's with the disgruntled group of former members who are seeking meaning in their spiritual journey. God seems to want me to be part of all of these groups of people as a voice of His message of mutual love and respect. I am not sure where I am being led but I know that God is the force within me and it as burning within me.

86

Inner Work

04/06/96 (Holy Saturday) - I Enter a Sports Stadium (dream)

Last night Joan, Grace and I had an interesting conversation. We covered many topics, but the underlying discussion was Saint Timothy's Lutheran Church and what's happening there now. Maybe this is the subconscious driving force behind last night's dream.

My dream begins as a friend and I enter a sports stadium. We are either attending the event at hand or pursuing someone or a group of people who are attending the game. I feel as if we are being watched constantly. I notice a small child or man leave by an upper exit and immediately several others follow after him. Then several others follow the other group out. My companion and I follow the two groups out into a large garage like area. It seems that the groups are preparing for a confrontation with each other. I notice one person hiding behind a pillar ready to jump out on a member of the other team and I grab him. He is holding a shotgun in his hands and I grab it also to prevent it from being used. He was going to attack the other group with it. I struggle with him and ask him if he would like me to use his weapon on him as I force the gun to point at his genitalia. The answer was an obvious frightened "NO! ". I collect all the members of both groups together in the middle of the room. Those on the side of the potential assailant grouped together opposite me while the to be victims stood behind me. I asked the assailant's group to identify themselves. They were hesitant at first but the weapon in my hand convinced them to announce their names and their belonging to a small gang of mischievous, not harmful, fun-loving sports fans. There seemed to be no reason for the presence of the gun I was holding except to start conversation. The group beside me were yet to be identified and I wondered what they were doing there. They seemed pleased that I was controlling the other group and forced them to identify themselves. I asked them who they were, but I received no answer until I said, "But what if the tide was turned and I was on this side of the room? " and I stepped beside the other group and pointed the gun at the unknown group. I asked them to identify themselves and each did so in turn stating their names and identifying themselves as FBI directors.

It was a peculiar bunch gathered there in that room my friend and I, 8 overzealous sports fans and 8 FBI directors but no small child that they originally pursued into the room. I asked the 8 FBI directors to mingle with the fans and become a cohesive group of 16. We, my friend and I, are now standing in the room in front of the 16 sitting at desks. I am reading a scripture lesson to them all and they look puzzled. The lesson quote that I remember stated that "A child shall lead them! " I mentioned to the group that I was glad that they were ready to accept their "Call". They all seemed amazed that such a disparate group as

87

they should be called together to follow God. It was noted that, as we have seen throughout the Bible, as God leads humankind the reverse happens when human leads human. A *child* "LED" the 16 into a room to bring them together through the conversation with another *older person* who "PURSUED" them into the room. I feel the "PULL" of God and the "PUSH" of humankind to get to that final connectivity with all souls is starting to come together in the world today. We, humankind, will not be able to resist the final "PULL" which is coming, and we will all be with God when the end finally comes.

05/08/96 - A Session with Bob (analysis)

A month has passed, and I finally set up a session with Bob Stoudt to review my dreams. I read my three dream entries from April and Bob probed my mind as to their meaning in my life today. It seems that I am constantly being torn internally with my struggle with vocation. I have yet to resolve the inner burning to spread the Word of God in a fashion that fulfills my desires. With all my work at Saint Timothy and with the dissidents who left I still feel a void in my vocational pull. More and more scriptures pass through my mind who new insight and clarity.

Christ's message to his disciples ("Who's sins you shall forgive they are forgiven and who sins you shall retain they are retained") keeps coming back to me. My mind's eye says that Christ was not just giving the disciples the gift of forgiveness, but He was announcing His desire for mankind to be more forgiving. We each should learn from Christ's life, be ever forgiving (it is difficult) and once forgiven release the pain and transgressions of those who offend you. Your inner self will feel full of God's grace and you will be at inner peace. The feeling of peace and tranquility realized from such gifting of forgiveness can only make one feel free; free of the anger and hurt caused by retained sins and transgressions. If you hold in the pain, anger and hate the only person who ultimately is hurt is yourself. The perpetrator of the pain and hurt has moved on in his or her life more likely than not while you are STUCK in your own muck and mire. The freedom of forgiveness is one of God's greatest gifts to us taught to us by Christ's life, death and resurrection.

Inner Work

06/07/96 - An Emerald Green Snake (dream)

One of those short but strange dreams. I meet a friend who has a basket in his arms. I open the basket and jump back slightly startled as a 4-foot-long snake uncoils from inside the basket. The snake is green (a bright emerald green to be exact). It crawls up my arm and wraps itself around me then slithers to the floor. I am alone facing the snake as it coils its tail and lifts itself upright, its head comes to about the middle of my chest. It tilts its head back and opens its mouth wide. I lean forward and put my head into its mouth and it swallows me whole. I now envision myself viewing the snake from a distance of about 10 feet. The snake is laying comfortably coiled on the ground with a large bulge (the swallowed me) in its middle. I am aware that I am inside the snake and feel very comfortable there. I awake wondering what the heck this dream means. I feel very much at peace upon awakening but confused about my dreams meaning.

06/27/96 - Joe Smith Dies

A friend, Joe Smith, at Xerox died yesterday of a heart attack. It was sudden and a surprise to all since Joe was only 38. I have taken time today to talk with several of his closest friends here and share with them my poem "*Musings on Death.* " I know there is a reason for me being where I am and maybe this sharing is part of it. More and more it seems God places me near people who need comfort in time of grieving. I can only hope that my gifts are a comfort to those I touch. God is always so near to us when we need comfort, all we have to do is accept his gentle touch.

08/27/96 - Dove
Frank J. Costanza

The world is never a lonely place
When believing in God's loving grace
The love that comes from God above
Free and graceful as the winging dove
Is a love given without a cost
To everyone found or lost.

Inner Work

10/30/96 - Letter to ACIM Believers

Hello fellow ACIM believers,

Allow me to introduce myself. My name if Frank James Michael Costanza, born 12/09/45 in Rutland, Vermont. I consider myself a Recovering Catholic and follower of the course in miracles since I was 13 (I know the course was not in text at that time, but the Holy Spirit touched me then and is with me every day). Allow me to explain, two years ago I started the course in miracles and realized that it fit in with how I had believed ever since I was 13 years old. Back in 1958 I was preparing myself for the priesthood by discussing possibilities with the Marist priests at Saint John DeMatha Catholic High School. I started attending mass daily at that time and felt a closeness to God that has never left me even though my religion path has wandered many ways since then. I struggled with the decision of whether to go into seminary or not and tested myself by joining the United States Marine Corps (a four-year stint). Two years (1965 and 1966) touring the beautiful country of Vietnam (unfortunately the war made it hard to see all the beauty) and watching mankind at its deadliest and ugliest allowed me to solidify my belief that God is within me and helps me through whatever life throws at me. Enough about the beginnings of my lifelong quest for what I found when taking the Course. I would like to be more in touch with other believers on the human as well as spiritual level. Please let me know how I become a part of your network. My e-mail address is either the one on this note (I am at work as a System Administrator at Xerox) or my home computer Internet address of PhoenixCI@gnn.com. PhoenixCI stands for our (my wife and I) consulting firm (Phoenix Collective Intelligence) rising from the ashes of our previous marriages. During the Course last year, the following quote appeared in my mind's eye and I keep it posted at my desk.

"WE ARE EACH BUT A SINGLE THREAD IN A TAPESTRY OF ILLUSION WOVEN ACROSS TIME BY EGO."

By the way the leader of my introduction to the course was Abigail Schearer. Thank you for allowing me this little dissertation.

12/11/96 - Directing a Construction Crew (dream)

Back to journalizing my dreams. Last night I dreamed I was at a house where I was directing a construction crew who were digging a new basement area. There were two areas being constructed on either side of a walkway that was half concrete then uneven asphalt to the road. The concrete section was to the left and the asphalt began in the middle of the new basement area. It seemed to be overlaying old concrete.

90

The new basement areas were poured concrete and ready for flooring to be put on top. Both sections had roughed in doorways on the left side. I remember commenting to Joan that the new areas provided a lot of storage area. The basement areas were at the rear of the existing structure and seemed to be for an addition or something. I had the crew tear up the asphalt section to replace it with concrete for consistency with the existing walkway. I noticed that under the asphalt was a previous concrete walkway that seemed to have collapsed into a sink hole or was eroded underneath by water washing away the soil. I told the crew to tear out the damaged areas and redo the walk. I also remember being asked to purchase a large area of land nearby for investment (100 acres). The person selling it said he needed to divest himself of the property for tax purposes, so he would sign the property over to me without exchange of moneys but when the profits were realized from sale of the produce grown on it he required me to give him half.

12/12/96 - Monday was My 51st Birthday

Monday was my 51st birthday (the top of the hill - maybe), my life has been hectic again probably due to my lack of listening to myself and keeping up with my dreams. I have registered for a retreat in April outside of San Francisco called Miracle Experience 13 "I Rest In God. " The retreat is sponsored by the California Miracles Center. I *found* this event while surfing the web looking for Course in Miracles contacts. The site is Mt. Alverno in Redwood City, CA (the foothills) and is run by Franciscan Sisters. I am very excited about this retreat and hope it will expand the ACIM work that I have been doing. For my birthday I received a pocket guide to the Nine Insights described in The Celestine Prophecy and an Experiential Workbook to the Celestine Prophecy. My work is beginning anew internally, and I must return to the regimen of the past and stop ignoring my unconscious self.

12/17/96 - A Large Dog Pawing (dream)

Strange dream, I saw a large dog pawing at an apartment building that seemed to have a narrower base than upper area. The dog was causing the building to teeter and I stopped him before he toppled it. The dog was larger than me and very friendly. I left the area and went into a lot where I found an old car for sale for $195. It looked pretty clean to me, so I asked the owner if it had been in a wreck recently because it was priced so low. I was thinking of buying it for my son who needs a car for work. When I got close to the car, I noticed that the roof was badly dented in as if the car had been rolled over in a wreck. I took it out for a test drive. It was VERY, VERY slow moving. It took half a block to get up to speed. I remember driving it near a railroad track and stood near it watching a slow-moving freight train pass. The train was pulled by an old-fashioned steam engine, big, black, large wheels, puffing billows of smoke and steam with its loud shrill steam whistle sounding. I woke up as the whistle screamed. It was 3:30 AM. I sort of half slept until I had to wake up for work pondering my last couple of dreams and what they could be telling me.

12/17/96 - Comments on my session with Bob (analysis)

Comments on my session with Bob today to discuss my dreams: We concentrated on this morning's dream. It contains three distinct venues. The first the interaction with the large dog. I described the dog to Bob as tall enough to paw the upper floor of the building. Bob asked me to see myself as the dog. I (the dog) am large and having fun pushing on this building, it's funny the way it wobbles when I push it. A man approaches and calls me a nice dog and asks me to stop pawing the building because I may topple it and hurt the occupants. I smile at the man and give him a big kiss (lick) and leave as he asked me to. The dog is a symbol of Asclepius (the healer) his significance in this dream seemed to be to alert me to the fact that something external (possibly our household) is causing me inner strife. I explained to Bob about the level of turmoil and stress present at home and he concurred that my psyche was trying to wake me up to what needs to be attended to. The big friendly dog is me and my pushing is to try to possibly topple the chaos in our home and the man (my external self) probably should have not stopped the dog from doing his task. This work ties in with my previous dream with the new foundations and large (100 acre) section of land that needs to be worked to grow produce with half the proceeds going back to the owner. This seemed to signify the I have a lot of work to do to get results and there is great cost (half of the profits) in the reaping of benefits. I intimated that this could be the task of bringing order to our chaotic household, a task that Joan and I have to work on together. Part of putting our house in order deals with my setting the example for Michael as he enters the world as an adult (the second vignette). The car I am looking at to help Michael get started is cheap and not very reliable (you get what you pay for). If I really wish to help Michael get started, I need to provide quality support and direction. Reduce the negative comments and attention to little annoyances and allow him to mature with a sense of care and compassion being directed at him not allusions of despair and hopelessness. This links to the third vignette (the freight train). Since it is a freight train it does not carry people rather other "STUFF" or a large "LOAD" (the tasks at hand within the household). It is also old (steam engine), slow moving, big and billowing (the wheels and smoke) and it got my attention (whistle "SCREAMING") and woke me up. My external self was made aware of my inner struggles. Psyche wanted my attention and got it fully.

12/29/96 - In a Large Dome Shaped Building (dream)

In a large dome shaped building. There are no seams visible on any walls inside or outside the dome is perfectly smooth as if made of acrylic or some type of plastic. The building is pure white in color with a circular opening in the middle of the floor with slides or chutes going down to a lower level. I walk to the railing to look down at the lower level. In the center of the lower level is a large blast furnace with openings near each chute (the end of the chute is about 2 feet from the furnace opening.) The furnace chimney goes straight up through the dome roof. I notice that the flames in the furnace are white hot, so hot that anything put into the furnace becomes instantly consumed. As I am standing there, workers come in carrying bodies on litters and push them down the chutes to cremate them. The technicians seem to take a tissue sample from each body before cremating them and places it into a small vial that is put in a small tube attached to the chute. As the body is sent down to the furnace the vial is also dropped down the tube to the lower level. The bodies slide down the chutes and sail across the gap into the furnace opening and are consumed by the flames almost instantaneously. The floor of the lower level seems to have a cloudy, gaseous substance flowing over it and as the vial entered the clouds a clone of the deceased is instantly generated. The clone is a perfect replica of the deceased and it would leave the area of the furnace by walking under the circular platform I was observing from. Once out of view I did not know where the clones went to. This process of cremation and instant rebirth seemed to go on continuously and no one seemed to notice my presence as an observer.

Inner Work

1997 DREAMWORK PROSE and POETRY

Overview of 1997

The year 1997 was a year of new turmoil. My spiritual direction seems to have taken off on a purely vertical path as my first dream intimates. I seem to bound towards the heavens and lose all connection with the horizontal. I have a sense of freedom from the present world of illusion that causes havoc in the world around me.

I start writing eulogies for friends' parents when the pass on to the next world and feel needed, or maybe the feeling is more a feeling of necessary rather than needed. My friends see me as a source of great comfort in their time of grief. My internal question is, "Is this my vocational call being answered? " The answer never seems to be fully answered but I feel changes within me that I cannot stop.

I begin to have dreams where I guide people from this "illusionary" world into the next world of "reality" where God opens His arms in love and forgiveness. I start to realize my potential as a healer and care giver.

Dream retreat #3 helps me cope with upcoming changes by helping to center me once again. Bob, as always, prods me into deeper work and exploration. My sense of inner peace is strengthened, and I move forward.

The second half of 1997 I once again became fully engaged in day to day existence and ignored my inner work. My ignorance of Psyche was not to last forever. As 1998 loomed on the horizon, Psyche was preparing a new barrage of dreams to keep me focused.

I am learning that I must constantly pay attention to myself and Psyche if I am to be comfortable with my life in the world of illusion.

Inner Work

01/12/97 - Driving with Joan to a Soccer Field (dream)

Driving with Joan to a soccer field where Mike left his soccer shoes. Parked the car near the first field and looked for Mike's shoes, they were not there. We walked up a path through the woods to another field to look for the shoes. When we neared the field, I realized we had left the keys in the car, so I went back to get them while Joan searched for the shoes. As I started down the wooded trail, I noticed that I could slide down the path without effort. My feet seemed to float a couple of inches above the ground. As the trail got steeper, I seemed to pick up speed and by moving left or right I could swing upwards into the sky as if I were on a large invisible swing going back and forth. When I reached a height where I was prone parallel to the ground below, I seemed to break free of the gravitation pull that brought me back down and I began floating in the clouds above observing the beautiful landscape below and the bright sunlit sky above. I seemed to be able to move around at will while floating in the clouds. It took no effort at all to glide around the sky. For a moment I felt a little panicky because I did not seem to be able to descend to the path below, but a feeling of inner warmth and calm came over me and I just enjoyed my freedom from the earth's grasp until my alarm woke me up.

Inner Work

02/17/97 - As Friends Depart
Inspired by the Death of Bill Supko

As we journey through our visit to the world of time and space our universe expands and contracts. At birth we know only a few special friends, mom, dad, siblings and the hospital personnel there at our time of entry into this life. As we grow our universe expands to include other relatives, neighbors, school acquaintances and casual social contacts near our home. This private universe which we create around us grows larger as we expand our knowledge and travels. Every now and then our universe changes size as a friend departs. This friend may move to another area, stop communicating with us for various reasons or perhaps leave our visible universe completely by death. As a child those departures are sometimes very painful until we learn how to cope with our changing world, eventually we learn to accept that which we cannot change even though we wish we could. Somewhere along the time and space continuum in which we journey we cross a point in which our universe begins the contract (or so it seems). We see more and more of our friends departing us by death than by movement within our universe. At this point our human vulnerability becomes more obvious to us and we start to search inward more for answers. If we allow ourselves to accept that our "visible" world is only a world of illusion created by our journey through and that all of creation (past, present and future) is God's perfect gift of love to us. And, as our soul takes its short journey through this phase which is framed by "our" constraints of time and place, we allow ourselves to learn from our journey and bring ourselves to a better understanding of "life" on this spaceship Earth. We then can accept the "losses" we experience with the knowledge that all of God's creation is one with God in universal light. Finally, through this knowledge, we can bring ourselves to inner peace, a peace that can only come from a God who totally loves His creation and does not condemn.

Inner Work

04/05/97 - *The Loss of a Parent*
by frank James Costanza

God touches each of our lives from birth to death. As we grow, we feel the touch of God (or as some refer to it; our Guardian Angel) many times. Most often we are not aware of that presence in our life as we brush it off as luck. Such as when we first learned to ride a bicycle and we teeter and almost fall but regain our balance and ride on. God, or the wing of our Guardian Angel, buoyed us up and protected us. Later on, we have many close calls with tough situations and God pulls us through. God helps us constantly by putting loving people in our lives: family, friends, lovers (Remember that first kiss?). Then there are the sadder moments when God touches our lives, those are the times when God calls one of those close to us to join Him in everlasting love and light. God reaches out and takes the hand of our loved one and they leave this world and go with God. We feel the pain of their departure and are saddened by the loss. We must rest assured and be happy, not sad, when God calls our loved ones away because they are now in a much better place full of love and peace. This is especially true when the one who departs is a parent. God put those special people in our lives for love and guidance and when God feels their job is done, He opens His arms and welcomes them with love. All we can do is say goodbye and find comfort in the fact that God loves all of His creation and will not condemn His children but bring them to everlasting peace. From this heavenly vantage point our parents can watch over us constantly and be there when we need them. All one needs to do is look inward at the God within and ask for help and He will provide whatever strength we require to get us through.

97

Inner Work

04/09/97 - Three Dreams

At a party or housewarming, many people present. Helping rearrange furniture for Linda Shearer. What appears to be a massive lightening flash occurs outside. We go outside to see and notice the night sky looks funny, areas of clouds with bright light behind. We see a couple sitting out looking also at the sky when a beam of light from the clouds envelopes them and they dissolve in the light and disappear. We walk and watch others go the same way until we are finally enveloped in light and go It is very peaceful in the light and we feel a great sense of love but several of us are returned to Earth. We tell of the peace and love felt and not to be afraid. I awake in my hotel room calm but bewildered. It is 1:20 AM so I go back to sleep.

Once again, I dream of the cloudy sky/with lights. They are more plentiful now and those of us who came back continue to tell others to not be afraid as the light will take them ro a place of great peace and love. I want to go back but I don't seem to be able to because my task is not done. Many areas now appear in the sky with multiple rays of light. The collection process is speeding up. I run and hug a friend as he enters the light and we disappear. I am once again sent back. I awaken, and it is 3 AM and I am facing the opposite way in the bed. I must get some sleep for work. I finally get back to sleep only to dream again.

05/15/97 – Larger Collection Areas (dream)

This time there are larger collection areas which seem to have platforms to step onto. I am again helping people to decide to go with the light. There seems to be more chaos around us, many are fearful but those who leave are full of happiness immediately. There are others like me on each platform with smiles of love and care on their faces helping people to step up and enter the light. I am standing with friends watching this all as the news broadcasts tell of great armies being amassed in several countries with a capacity of mass destruction. The collection process is speeding up to save the faithful for many are called but few are chosen as many refuse to take the final step into the light. I am stepping into the light to leave as all hell breaks loose on Earth. I leave with an awareness that those left behind will be engulfed in a devastating war that will destroy them all. I also feel a great outpouring of love from the light that will bring them all to eternal peace after the great cataclysm is fulfilled. I wake up exhausted. It is 6 AM and I must get ready to go to work. I can still feel the anxiety I felt because I could not go into the light at a time of my choosing. Not in

98

my time but in God's time I say to myself and I am at inner peace.

07/08/97 - A Coven of Witches (Dream)

I am lying in bed in a simple room (bed, table and a chair). Seven women come in and one speaks to me saying that they were a coven of witches and that I was to make love to each of them this night. They were each to bear a female child from their bonding with me. I tell the leader (I assumed the one speaking was their leader) that in all my relationships I have only produced male children and since the male is the genetic link to a child's sex, I felt it unlikely that all, if any, of them would have female children. She said that it would happen as she said and then I noticed I was naked in bed and the first of the seven was on top of me making love to me. This continued until all seven were satisfied the last being the leader who totally exhausted me with her sexual antics. They all left together, and I woke up exhausted in my simple room. NOTE: In my view witches are not evil women but gifted.

Inner Work

07/11/97 – WERNERSVILLE DREAM RETREAT 3
Being Taught to use Calipers (Dream)

Getting to sleep was difficult this night because I was soaking in the peacefulness of this Holy place in Wernersville, PA. I finally sleep and dream of being shown how to use calipers to measure things and how to use special pliers to open and attach spring clips. I awake wondering why I needed instruction in something so familiar to me as hand tools I had used in the past.

07/12/97 - A Gap in My Oak Tree 9:30 AM

I sit in the shade looking at my great oak tree and notice a gap in the branches where the limbs are dead. A bird sits on the highest dead branch and sings a beautiful song to welcome the day.

07/12/97 - A Session with Bob 10:15 AM (dream analysis)

I meet with Bob to discuss my dreams. We poke around for meaning then the discussion turns to the present status of my career. A two-and-a-half-year contract ends next week. A new product, TRAV-L-CISE, has been developed by me and is moving forward. A potential new job with HP looms on the horizon to establish a global help desk for their products. The next two months seem to be destined to be full of anxiety, challenge, unsure futures and trust in God. My relearning old skills could be the job at HP doing something I did almost twenty years ago in IBM I know my abilities but am apprehensive at the prospect of attaching myself again to the corporate world. My new product, TRAV-L-CISE, opens a whole new world of possibilities. The exercises center on the abdomen and release of stress and strain. The connection can be made to the seven witches (strong feminine symbols) and female offspring (a new endeavor for me). The lead witch proclaims it will happen. The choice will be up to me and I stand at the fork in the road. Which way is the way of ego which will return me to the fork to make the choice again and which is the way of Holy Spirit who leads me to future growth and development. The choice will be mine to make in the near future. This weekend of self-centering will help me prepare for my future in this illusionary world. I can feel the nearness to the "Holy Instant", that point in our time bound world in which the present always is and time is meaningless. That place where we are one with God and all of creation. A place of total love and peace. I can feel the rapture within welling up and pouring forth to all humanity. God is Love, God's in me, Love is all that I can be.

100

Inner Work

07/12/97 - Preparing for Eucharist 11:00AM

A silent moment preparing for Eucharist. Soft music plays as people slowly fill the chairs in silence, smiles are shared. Father Jack Barron presides, the sermon on dealing with fear touches all. Communion is shared after peace is shared. Father Barron hugs me after the service, a friend for the past several years with a great heart.

07/12/97 - Lunch in Silence 1:00PM

Lunch in silence, just smiles of love and peace shared. Back to my room for a nap (these retreats are exhausting as your mind works hard). My body seems extremely tired today. I sleep without dreams, I awake with a date in my mind February 13, 1937. I sense it was a Sunday, but I do not know its significance. I must research it.

07/12/97 - A Brief Respite 4:30PM

A brief respite from mental work as I work on a jigsaw puzzle for relaxation before dinner.

07/12/97 - A Bountiful Dinner 5:15PM

A bountiful dinner in silence, everyone looks so full of peace. After dinner a silent search of the book store finds a neat book "Hidden Women of the Gospels" which I purchase. I go to my room to peruse my book It is 9PM and I have finished half of the book and my eyes are heavy. A shave and a ritual bath and I am ready for a good night's rest after a box of Frosted Flakes.

07/13/97 - A Bengal Tiger 1:20AM (dream)

In the woods behind a housing development, Tony and a friend are playing with a pet monkey. I am watching them having fun and tell them it is time to bring their pet home when I notice a large rope net stretched across an area to my right like a trap used in a jungle. Beyond the net, I notice a large Bengal tiger crouched in the bushes. I yell to Tony not to go that way to avoid the net and the tiger. We head off to our left to leave the woods as the tiger starts to follow us. I yell to Tony to move faster but don't run to get out of the woods. He picks up the pace as the tiger moves closer. As we leave the woods a man is in his garden in the back yard in front of us and I warn him of the

101

tiger. He looks up and top his left and sees the tiger coming towards him. Tony starts running through the fenced in yards to home as the tiger is distracted. I walk slowly toward the fence gates as the tiger slowly follows me. As I reach our back yard, I yell to Jean to get the kids inside for protection. The tiger is not far behind me as a young boy starts out into the street which attracts the animal's attention. Jean rushed out of the back yard to chase the tiger as I rush in the house to call 911 for assistance. I yell at Jean to keep away from the tiger before I enter the house. I notice that the young boy had taunted the animal and was mauled by the tiger as Jean chased it away. I was on the phone pleading with the 911 operator to hurry as the tiger entered the house leaving a path of bloody paw prints in its wake. It cornered me in the kitchen (phone still in my hand talking to 911) and softly pawed my hand down and started licking my fingers like a large house cat would. It was sucking on my fingers as I was telling 911 not to use sirens and I woke up. The sensation of my hand in the cat's mouth remained vivid.

1998 DREAMWORK PROSE and POETRY

Overview of 1998

The year is 1998 and I continue to grow and dream. The spiritual depth of my dreams seems to be expanding. I have to continually remind myself to avoid an inflated feeling of the Ego. My struggles with everyday life deepen as I try to remain within the illusionary world around me. I know I am avoiding my call for ministry as I view ministry but the economic realities around me and my strong sense of family responsibility cause me conflict. My dreams at night push me toward a different vocation while my time when awake play heavy on my psyche. My sense is that I am still in the tumultuous throws of male menopause, a struggle I thought I was through.

Dream Retreat #4 is fantastic, Bob's opening session takes us into active imagination an I seem to sense where Bob is taking us before he speaks. Phaedra comes to me and lifts me up and prepares me for the retreat. My "dream partner" for this retreat is Sandy Patton, a friend from church who is interested in dream work. We shared a ride to the retreat and our discussions helped prepare us for our silence and dreams.

The retreat helps me visualize the "vertical" and "horizontal" components of my life. In a dream I named "I Discover Myself" I find myself and an answer to my vocational "call". As usual, my dreamwork leaves me full of wonder at God's presence in my life.

I close the inner work section of this book in July of 1998 as my dreams become more and more consumed with Biblical meaning and prophecy. I promise Psyche that I will continue to listen to and journal my dreams.

Inner Work

01/03/98 - A Forestry Station in the Woods (Dream)

A new year and strange dreams. I am in a forestry station in the woods of the great Northwest Territory. There are three others with me. One, who is the leader, has a pager and is responsible for reacting to any fire calls in the area with his team. We seem to be engrossed in games of some sort and we leave to go to the small town nearby. Everyone asks why we haven't responded to the fire on the mountain and our leader checks his pager, sure enough he had been called but he did not hear the page. Perhaps we were all enjoying ourselves too much and made too much noise, but it didn't seem to matter. The fire in the mountains did no damage at all it just glowed, and flames leapt high, but nothing was consumed. (I get a short glimpse of a game using magnetically controlled images.) We go into a public bathroom. It is large with open holes in the floor similar to Japanese toilets with pull drapes around each like in hospital emergency rooms. One of my companions says to me that there is a body in one of the toilets. I look and all you can see are the persons arched back protruding from the hole in the floor. It is as if he dove into the hole with his head, hands and feet down. I wake up only to half consciousness before I drift back into another more pleasant dream. This dream is almost prosaic and fills me with great love as my goddess returns.

02/28/98 – My Goddess Returns (dream)

The crisp autumn air of the great northwest forest teases my senses. The smell of pine and fresh fallen leaves fills the air. The sun is setting with a reddish glow as the northern lights dance happily in the sky above. She opens her cabin door and stands there half clothed, only a shirt covers her creamy soft white flesh. She invites me in. The soft warm glow of many candles lights the room with licks of dancing flames. She excuses herself to get the rest of her clothes on as I enter her home. The sweet smell of candle wax fills my nostrils as she returns to me and we embrace. Her body feels wonderful in my arms as I kiss her softly on her cheek. We had been in each other's thoughts earlier that day, so the embrace felt fulfilling. The candle light dances in her beautiful red hair as I look at her. Her youthful body feels wonderful against my overweight and tiring older frame. Her touch makes me feel younger and more invigorated as I realize that this short embrace is just a gift of love to waken my youthful soul. I dream of holding her forever, but my visit is to be short. I must leave this heavenly place, this room full of love, and return to the illusionary world my soul committed itself to. We embrace once more as I leave, the sensuous smell of her body mingles with the sweet smell of the candles

104

as I say goodbye. Perhaps another time I will be able to stay and leave the chaotic world of illusion behind and enjoy her loving embrace forever. I awake feeling an emptiness in my heart.

03/17/98 - In a Military Vehicle (dream)

In a military vehicle near an airstrip, many people being evacuated from the area to avoid the upcoming conflagration. I am in civilian clothes and get out of the vehicle to direct people to the aircraft for their flight out. As the last person boards the aircraft, I bid them safe passage and I return to the road near the airstrip. I am not to leave the area only see that the others safely depart. I awake as the opposing military personnel gather around me from all directions. I do not feel threatened by their presence.

03/18/98 - A Room with a Large Couch (dream)

Two unusual dreams, first I am in a room with a large couch with many people seated on it. Each person has a newborn baby in their arms that they are dedicated to care for. I feel a great affinity to each and every one of the babies. There are people in front of the room simultaneously teaching all the babies how to count in all the major languages of the world: one is saying ein, sweigh; another one, two; another uno, duo and so on. I am teaching Japanese counting ichi, ni, san, shi. I am explaining the simplicity of the Japanese counting system to all. I go over to hold and cuddle each of the babies and show them my love for them. After I have held each the dream abruptly ends/changes and I am in a wilderness area on a finger of land near a bend in a great river. Behind me is a great chasm with beautiful forested land I am sitting in some bleachers with several people looking toward the river watching a group of loggers or woodsmen clearing trees and brush around the river's edge. I know I have watched this scene many times before each time with new observers and a different crew working the woods at the river's edge. As the woods become more stripped of its natural beauty the river comes down the gorge to the bend in a great wave and engulfs all of us in the great wave cleansing the finger of land of all those who were desecrating the river. Two other observers and I grip the earth as the wave passes over us with all the logs and others washing the impurities into the chasm behind us. We stand there in amazement as we see the finger of land has been returned to its pristine state. To our left at the tip of the finger of land is a large building in front of which a fourth survivor stands. He seems to exude love and understanding. I awake realizing that the building he was in front of is the place where the children were being taught.

06/07/98 - Taking an Exam from Bob Stoudt (dream)

Taking an exam from Bob Stoudt, there are 4 students in the class including me. On my desk is a radiator and 4 fittings, I am to pick which one came off object on my desk and describe soldering or welding technique used. Easy to do by turning radiator over and only one fitting had same shape flange. Looked for paper and pencil. Pencil was unsharpened. Pencil sharpener was in pieces, had to hold together to push pencil in and twist pencil to sharpen it. Borrowed paper from Bob and started to write. I began 1/3 the way down and was writing about a beautiful cat in front of me. I wrote first line, then the title one line above, then the date one line above that and finally my name on the top line. Went back to where the pencil sharpener was and the whole area was cordoned off and I was not allowed to pass. As I looked past the barrier the area beyond was completely empty like a void. I turn around and there are no desks anymore just a large table where Bob is teaching how to prepare a turkey for cooking. On the table is a large turkey carcass, large enough for me to crawl into to help season the insides. Bob starts to salt the bird as I crawl out and pick up a tomahawk to carve the turkey. It looked like the tomahawk of Sean's I found in the car trunk. Bob took the tomahawk and stuck it into the table top and led Tony and I into a storage room on the left to pick out some materials to construct a holding pen in the back yard for kittens. There must have been a dozen new kittens still bloody from birth in the pen. Tony was teaching them to eat while we watched from outside the fence, sitting with a group of beautiful women in the grass listening to a lecture. The woman next to me is asking if someone would go get a soda for her, no one volunteers so she gets on her unicycle to go get it herself. I ask her to get one for me also and she leers at me and rides off. We are all in a set of bleachers and a man is selling snowballs and asking each of us which flavor we want. Everyone wants a different combination of very exotic fruit flavors. He stops taking orders when he gets to the 4 of us whom were in the original class as the scene shifts again. This time we are in a car following some people until they make a left turn towards a covered bridge. I make a U-turn to go back as the occupants of the other car laugh at us and call us chicken. We return to the driveway and drive towards the door which opens, and we drive through the house to the back yard. It looks like there is a petting zoo there with lots of people milling around. I wake up actively remembering all the events and drifting in and out of each scenario.

Inner Work

06/20/98 – 1998 DREAM RETREAT 4
Wernersville, PA
Evening Session

Bob opens our retreat with a review of the process of searching for the healing dream with the newcomers. As always, I attend this first session to assist in my preparation for the weekend. This retreat Bob tries something new in our group opening session. We bring a pillow from our rooms and lay on the floor as Bob plays a tape of the ocean and soft music. He talks quietly to us to have us look inward in preparation for our silence. As I look inward at my ocean setting, slow curling waves lapping at my feet, white salty foam caressing my tired body, I drift from scene to scene of my times at the beach in my life. My focus comes to rest on my first honeymoon to Ocean City, Maryland. Doris and I are sitting on the beach as I notice a young girl (18 - 20) sitting on the boardwalk looking troubled, a sad puppy dog look on her face. I feel her need for comfort as I stare at her pained expression. Doris walks away for 20 - 30 minutes then comes back. I did not notice her leaving and she is angry that I am still staring at the troubled child. I focus on my "dis-ease" I brought with me "I need to be better understood. " As I drift deeper into thoughts and see myself slowly die and decompose I feel a great weight lift from my soul. As I become a bare skeleton I feel a presence and a woman appears in intense white light. It is Phaedra, my goddess, as she leans down to caress my skeleton and lift me up Bob starts to talk about someone being there to put my body to rest. As I return to center and awareness my hands are numb and my body feels light. I am relaxed and ready for my retreat. Phaedra is here as my companion this weekend and I feel loved.

06/21/98 – 05:45 AM – A Night Without Dreams

A night without dreams that I recall. It took a while to fall asleep last night. I could not put my mind to rest. Short snippets of memories kept me awake as if I were reviewing my life and my relationships. Nothing stayed in my mind for more than a fleeting moment. I finally succumb to sleep and rest peacefully. I woke up at 4 AM with no dreams to recall. I lay there pondering my "dis-ease" I brought with me. I need to be better understood by those around me. No one knows how I deal with pain and anger because they cannot comprehend or accept my concept of total forgiveness. I drift back to sleep as Phaedra caresses my brow. I awaken at 05:45 dreamless again but much warmer and moist from nocturnal emission. If I dreamt it was fulfilling but I have no recollection of any dreams last night.

107

Inner Work

06/21/98 – 06:00 AM

EZEKIEL 37

The hand of the LORD came upon me, and he carried me out by his spirit and put me down in a plain full of bones. He made me go to and fro across them until I had been round them all; they covered the plains countless numbers of them, and they were very dry. He said to. me, "Man, can these bones live again? " I answered, "Only thou knowest that, Lord GOD. " He said to me, "Prophesy over these bones and say to them, 0 dry bones, hear the word of the LORD. This is the word of the Lord GOD, to these bones: I will put breath into you, and you shall live. I will fasten sinews on you, bring flesh upon you, overlay you with skin, and put breath in you, and you shall live; and you shall know that I am the LORD. " I began to prophesy as he had bidden me, and as I prophesied there was a rustling sound and the bones fitted themselves together. As I looked, sinews appeared upon them, flesh covered them, and they were overlaid with skin, but there was no breath in them. Then he said to me, "Prophesy to the wind, prophesy, man, and say to it, These are the words of the Lord GOD: Come, 0 wind, come from every quarter and breathe into these slain, that they may come to life. " I began to prophesy as he had bidden me: breath came into them; they came to life and rose to their feet, a mighty host.

I open the folded sheet Bob handed us after last night's session and read it. The passage from Ezekiel touched me as the memory of our group collectively imagining themselves dying and decomposing until only our bones remained. We then were laid to rest and resurrected to a new experience, this dream retreat.

I go outside for a short walk. I stop at the statue of the Sacred Heart of Jesus and say a short prayer. I look at my oak tree from all sides. It is strong and full of life. I sit in the grass drinking in the early morning rays of sunlight and watching small birds flit in and out of the boughs of my great oak. I listen to the varied songs of the morning. There once was a time long ago when I was able to identify each songbird by its song but now I just sit and peacefully listen to God's chorus in the trees. The sky is so beautiful this morning, bright blue with fluffy white clouds drifting overhead. The hills and valleys shining emerald green in the early morning sun laced with dewdrops, small crystals of moisture lightly dancing on the tips of each blade of grass. The fragrance of the evergreen shrubs around the novitiate tantalize the sense of smell beckoning one to soak in all that is around them and become one with the earth. To feel that inner peace, that gift from God that can never be taken away. My soul is enriched each time I visit this Holy place and, through silence, hear the voice of God through His creation around me. I know that God understands and loves me and I am at peace with myself.

06/21/98 – 08:30 AM – A Reading on the Sacred Heart of Jesus

I left a note for Bob this morning attached to a small booklet I picked up and read on the *Sign of Salvation, The Sacred Heart of Jesus*. My note read:

> Bob, you might enjoy this pamphlet. It addresses the "cultic" nature of Saint John's sign and talks of the bronze serpent.
> Frank

06/21/98 – 09:30 AM – Another Peaceful Walk

The end of another peaceful walk among the trees, flowers and blackberries. Squirrels scurrying about, woodpeckers knocking on the trees, birds and insects chirping happily. It is a gorgeous day. As I return to the novitiate, I nod hello to Sandy Patton, my dream partner this weekend. Her expression looks as if she could use a hug and for a moment I consider walking over and giving her one. I pass up the urge in order to avoid breaking the solitude of our retreat process. Sandy is a young woman from church who I shared a ride with to Wernersville. She's a member of our adult discussion group and friend of both Joan and me. Our conversations en route helped me better focus on my retreat goals. I sit in a comfortable chair by the window and enjoy the gentle breeze of God's breath across my brow. I am eating a delicious orange and contemplating last Sunday's adult discussion group. At dinner before the retreat, Sandy was eating a lemon slice and we discussed eating the rind of citrus fruits. I told her how our children think I am strange because I eat an orange as they eat an apple, rind and all. Sandy walked by and noticed I was eating the orange, rind and all, and smiled hello to me. I am recalling that Marian LeFevre made note of the strength of my vertical self (inner connection with God) and applauded it but questioned why I have little, if any, horizontal attachment (connection with the duality of life.) I finally come to realize that it is my studies of theology, *A Course in Miracles*, major religions of the world and Christ's teachings on forgiveness that allow me to remain in the vertical with little or no horizontal. I truly believe in the "Divine Instant" or that moment of pure present (viewing the "present" as God's gift) where there is no past or future only inner vertical connection with God. As I continue to stay within that "Divine Instant" there is no horizontal as time is of no consequence only connectivity with one's spiritual center, the Pure Vertical. As I stay centered the world of duality around me has less and less pull on me and the power of forgiveness strengthens my resolve. My "need" for understanding, my "dis-ease" I brought with me this weekend to search for inner help can only be satisfied if I remain centered. I know I have an inner calling to teach my belief in total forgiveness to those who would listen. I also am gaining an insight into how my call is to be (or is being) fulfilled. Over the last several years, I have discussed with many people; family close friends and even strangers, this inner call I have felt. Joan and I had a tearful discussion on the possibility that sometime in the future I may need to move on in my calling to teach others Christ's message of forgiveness. Yesterday at dinner before arriving at Wernersville Sandy Patton and I had a lengthy discussion on our upcoming dream retreat and our individual life struggles. Sandy noted that my deep feelings of a call may be difficult for Joan to handle on some levels. I related last Sunday's adult discussion to Sandy as she was absent. I took my thoughts, feelings, hopes and dreams into this retreat of silence and, all though I have yet to recall a dram, exclusive of the opening session's "active imagination" with Phaedra, I now feel that my call *is* being filled on a daily basis with my practicing what I preach concerning forgiveness. My participation in the adult discussions, even though small in attendance, is a filling of my inner call in a way that I never recognized nor gave credence to before. My call is to teach, through example, Christ's love and forgiveness every day to each person I come into contact with. My thoughts of fulfillment of my call later in life were erroneous and a means of escaping the reality of my struggle with horizontal. There is no past or future only the "Divine Instant" where time is nonexistent, and we are one with God. I have taken another leap in my faith journey. I know I will always struggle with the duality of life in the world of illusion, but my vertical strength will pull me through. God loves me and has once again gifted me with a Divine Insight. Life is wonderful. I return to my room and find a note from Bob attached to the pamphlet I left him to peruse.

His note read: Frank, Thanks for the chance to look at this. Some interesting points B including the bronze serpent ' Christ one.   Bob

06/21/98 – 01:00 PM – Session with Bob

Bob congratulates me on my growth and the revelations I felt concerning myself. My realization is that I must stay connected with the horizontal and grounded while remaining spiritually vertical. Identifying my "call" has helped finalize my transition of the last few years. We discuss my handling of pain and anger and forgiveness. Bob applauds

110

my method of recognizing the anger, taking ownership of its pain and then pushing it off to my higher self and God. He defined my process as very Buddhist in nature and obviously healthy and cleansing. I hope my notes from this retreat will help others to understand my "dis-ease" with their skepticism and allow them to be gifted by the power of my "call" to teach through example. I do not wish for people to perceive of me as having a holier-than-thou attitude. I only ask for understanding and acceptance of the fact that it is "*MY*" process. It is not necessary for them to be like me but to feel my love for all people and things for what it is: a pure gift of love and grace from God, a gift we each have been endowed with from birth. We are all God's children and as such we are loved, cared for and forgiven beyond belief.

06/21/98 – 04:45 PM – An Interesting Dream

Laid down after a long walk when finished with lunch and fell asleep, a long restful sleep. Woke up from an interesting dream. I was in a small hotel room with Joan and I am getting ready to go play softball. I searched through a stack of gloves for mine but could not find it. I ran out to the field to play hoping to find my glove there. I was the third man in the batting order, but I still had not found my glove. A friend says I left it in the coach's office in the school building at the other side of the fields. The fields consist of four softball diamonds and I must run through the bleacher areas to get to the building. I must hurry as the first batter for my team is at the plate. As I run he hits a long home run into the farthest field. I run toward the building and notice that I am high above the fields on the edge of a cliff looking down at the players. I get to the building and must run through classrooms and the gymnasium to get to the office. As I enter the gymnasium there is a cycling event taking place and I must run through the cyclists to get to the other side. The cyclists are racing fast but seem to be flat on the floor. I must dodge their fast spinning wheels and handlebars on the floor as I traverse the center of the room. I finally reach the coaches office and he hands me my glove. I turn to leave back the way I came when I woke up.

111

Inner Work

Personal notes on my dream:

- The large pile of gloves I searched through were in many sizes but none fit
- I obviously left for the game unprepared to participate
- No one seemed to care that I needed to find my glove
- As I ran the flat field edges became high cliffs with me running on top looking down at the horizontal fields below
- I had to run a maze of rooms to get to my destination
- In the gymnasium I was completely vertical while all the cyclists were racing around horizontally
- I had a difficult time traversing the floor dodging all the horizontal wheels and spokes spinning at my feet
- When I finally picked up my glove, the object of my quest, the dream ended

Inner Work

06/21/98 – 05:45 PM – A Request for Bob

Left a note for Bob to see if he had time to discuss my dream this evening. Dinner was, as usual, delicious. I sat across from Sandy this evening. It is unusual that with all the people at these retreats you rarely run into others as you walk the grounds. It seems as if God directs us each in our own journey and only allows contact if necessary. The soft music playing makes dinner relaxing. Sandy is a good person and a friend who finds it hard to believe that I will actually be silent for any time much less a whole retreat. A distant roll of thunder announces an impending storm.

06/21/98 – 06:00 PM – A Short Note to Sandy

Sandy,
    A short note of thanks for sharing the ride to this retreat with me. Our conversation was enjoyable and thought provoking and dinner was delightful. Now that you "KNOW" that I can be silent when necessary I hope our friendship will continue to grow in spirituality. Last week's adult discussion and our dinner conversation helped in making this retreat one of great discovery for me. It is a blessing to have such strong women friends around me to help me grow and feel my inner self. Joan will be glad to know that I realize now that my "call" is being filled daily. Thanks again.
God's love, Frank

Inner Work

06/21/98 – 06:15 PM – Bob Makes Extra Time for Me

Bob makes extra time for me to review my dream of discovery. As we grasp the essence of my dream Bob asks me to put a title on it. I come up with several in my mind but what sticks is "I reach my quest's goal" but then I change it to "I Discover Myself. " Psyche, throughout the dream prevented me from getting in the game by placing obstacles in my way; no glove, unprepared, left the lineup to search for my glove, high cliffs above the horizontal fields below, grounded to a surface full of horizontal obstacles (cyclists and spinning wheels), etc. Finally, when I get my glove and am ready to return to the game, Psyche awakens me to prevent me from playing. Psyche is making me aware of the need to stay grounded and be in touch with the horizontal, human reality as I see it in the world of illusion. Psyche does not tear down my vertical strength only makes me aware of the horizontal around me that I must reconnect with; family, friends, relationships, etc. Without that connectivity my "call" cannot continue to be filled and I will become out of touch, overly engrossed with the vertical. Bob gives me the example of the absent-minded professor who is so engrossed in his tasks that he cannot see the world around him. This reminded me of Albert Einstein who was at the University of Maryland for while years ago. One of my engineering professors had known and worked with him back then. He related a story of Einstein working so hard on a project that he spent days lost in thought and his friends and colleagues had to come to his room periodically to remind him to eat. In a similar way I have allowed the vertical growth to consume me of late and I must now become better grounded or risk losing all that is around me.

Inner Work

06/21/98 – 07:00 PM – Sandy Left a Note for Me

I return to my room to find a note from Sandy Patton. Sandy wrote:
Frank,

    It still amazes me at times how things happen . . . I feel blessed to be sharing this time and space with you. Your name (or whatever you represent to me) has been appearing in my journal. For that, I am thankful that we were able to share this together. Perhaps someday I will be able to explain more fully how your presence has impacted me.

    Meanwhile, I am glad this retreat is a time of discovery for you . . . I am finding much joy and peace in this time. Don't know if I had the "big dream" yet, but I sure had an annoying one . . . I had sex with Ricky Ricardo!! Met with Bob and he helped me get it in perspective, and it somehow fits my theme for this weekend (relationships, intimacy . . All that fun stuff!!)

    And yes, DP, I guess I was initially surprised at your silence, but maybe not so much anymore . . . now that I'm beginning to know you differently.
Peace, Sandy

06/21/98 – Midnight

I wake from a dream and go the bathroom. I return to my room and lay back in bed recalling the dream. Laying there not writing in my journal as I will write it down when I get up in the morning because I am tired and want to go back to sleep. Psyche won't let me fall asleep until I put my dream to paper. It is now 01:30 AM as I write. I am in the American Legion bar buying a drink. I scatter my pocketful of change on the bar to count out the exact change even though in the pile of change there are several plastic chits that I could pay for the drink with. Standing there as a friend stops by to say hello and the scene shifts to our home office. Several of the PCs are missing (the best ones) and I go into the house to find my son and his friends. They are using the PCs to set up a game room to play in. I ask them to return the PCs and they start carrying them back to the office. As they carry them I notice that the outer cases are not there (they were when I walked in the room). Also, the boys are not being careful with the systems as they carry them. I ask them to be careful and they bring the rest back to the office. As I check out each system I back up all the data to tape for security. I take the tapes to the office next door for the security company to protect them. I ask them to be sure the data is safe, and the security person opens a drawer beneath his chair (literally underneath the seat of his chair) and throws the tapes in with a grin. My confidence is not buoyed by this laissez faire attitude, but it will have to do. I return to the office and survey the area as I wake up.

115

Inner Work

06/22/98 – 06:00 AM – A Beach Dream

I lay in bed for a long time trying to capture details of my dream, but it still remains fragmented. I am at a beach with a friend. His daughter is playing in the surf in an inner tube. Each wave seems to toss her back to the wave behind until she is three or four waves out then she rides in on the next wave. This continues as my friend and I talk about the commercial development at the shore. He does not like all the new restaurants nearby as they clutter the view of the beach he loves so much. He comments on the mediocre food they serve as we listen to his little girl's gleeful laughter in the surf. The scene shifts, and I am parking in a lot near one of the newer restaurants. It is pouring rain and I am soaked. I walk to the covered entrance to meet three women friends who are getting out of a Rolls Royce. The one who was driving lost an election bet to the other two and had to rent the car and treat them to dinner. One of them said I had some mail at the house down the street from Peggy McDaniels, an old friend from my Young Republican days. She was Miss Mississippi Young Republican at the 1975 YR Leadership Conference when I met her. I walked down the beach in the pouring rain until I reached the beach house. I walked up the stairs into the house to pick up the mail. The top of the stairs was above the handrail, so I had to climb down the furniture to reach the center of the room. Water was pouring off my hair and clothes all over the furniture as I went in. As I picked up the mail I seemed perfectly dry. I open the large envelope from Peggy and it is a printing from a magazine ad showing her in a chef's hat, a pinafore and apron with a spatula in one hand and a cook book in the other. She is a renowned cook on a public television station, I wake up.

06/22/98 – 09:30 AM – Pierre Teilhard de Chardin

After breakfast I stopped in the library to look up Pierre Teilhard de Chardin since Father George Williams had a quote of his outside his room that touched me on several levels. I found "Hymn of the Universe" in the library and started to glance at his writings but his words consumed me, and I read it all. He, in the 1920's to 1950's was experiencing the same feelings and understanding of Christ's love and forgiveness as I. The quote that George had framed read: Some day after we have mastered the winds, the wave, the tides and gravity we will harness for God the energies of love and then for the second time in the history of the world man will have discovered fire.

116

Inner Work

06/22/98 – 09:30 AM -A Final Walk

I take final walk to breathe in this Holy place.

06/22/98 – 02:00 PM – A Fulfilling Retreat

This has been another wonderfully fulfilling retreat experience. I leave feeling blessed again.

06/22/98 – 03:00 PM – Closing Goodbyes

We all gather one final time to review the retreat experience with each other. Not much is shared only brief comments on fulfillment and hugs of goodbye. Sandy and I head for her car and out of silence. Decompression will be difficult this week.

06/26/98 – A Dream of Revelation

I awaken from a dream that can only be described as one of revelation, Biblical revelation. I felt a sense of oneness with the dimension of time and I was being taught and being given a vision of the second coming of God. My teacher was reminding me of the birth and life of Jesus Christ and how His own people, the Jews, denied who He was. They were expecting a great King and Leader to destroy their enemies and give them power but what they received was a great teacher of God's Love and Grace. I was shown how Christians today are expecting the second coming of God to be the physical return of Jesus Christ to gather up His people and let the rest of the world be damned. I was then given a review of the last century and the evolution of man toward a more global community. The history lesson included both world wars, Korea, Vietnam, Bosnia, a glimpse of all the wars and struggles of the many nations of the world. I was given a review of the reunification of humanity (the reversing of the tower of Babel) through scenes of positive change such as; the tearing down of the Berlin Wall, the removal of the Iron Curtain, the opening of the Bamboo Curtain, the breakup of the Soviet Union, the reunification of Germany, the new peace in Ireland, the Ecumenical movement, the exploration of space and myriads of other glimpses of the world wide peace process. I was taught that the second coming was not a return to this world of the human entity of Jesus Christ rather the evolution of the Children of God into a world-wide body filled with love for one another. The second coming is to be the tearing down of the walls (barriers) put up between people by organized religion that makes claims that they are right and everyone else is wrong. "Come to MY church because we know God

117

better that the others do. " God is coming again like Christ did as He threw the money changers out of the temple and turned religion of 2000 years ago on its head. Only this time His coming is through all of humanity, Father/Mother God will return through the hearts and minds of all of us as we evolve spiritually. The divisions between religions will fall. Christians, Jews, Moslems, Buddhists, Hindus, Mystics, Native Americans, any and all people of any belief or non-belief will come to understand that there is but one Mother/Father God and that God belongs to no one group, sect, cult, religion or whatever kind of division or walls humans try to put up between themselves. God is the love and grace within all of God's creation the holds the whole of creation together. Without God there would be nothing. Our new beginning (the second coming) is in process now and will evolve faster and faster as modern technology makes communications faster and faster. Languages will no longer be barriers as computers will be able to instantly translate for each of us. The electronic impulses within the computer circuitry is like microscopic tongues of flame of the Holy Spirit touching each and every one of us as the Internet connects the Global Village from pole to pole, east to west, planet to planet and universe to universe.

06/29/98 – A Dream of Giving Food Away

I awaken from a dream where I am on the seventh floor of a building displaying new inventions that were developed in the lab I was in. In the lab there is a refrigerator/freezer that we a filling with beef (steaks, roasts etc.). As we are putting platter after platter of the meat in more platters appear, there seems to be no end to the quantity of meat being stored. I take a platter with me as I leave the lab to go to the rest room. As I leave the lab I notice the wall in front of me is being renovated, I try to push through the layer of insulation to get to the other side, but I can't. I go to a door to the right which has no knob on it and push it open to enter the hall. There is no rest room on this floor, so I take the elevator down to the first floor, platter in hand. The elevator door opens to a pristine shopping mall located on the first floor of the building. As I look for the rest room people passing by take the steaks from the platter in my hands. No matter how many they take the platter never seems to become empty. I find the rest room and place the platter on a table next to the door as I go in to use the facilities. As I finish washing my hands and leave the rest room I pick up the still overflowing platter and return to the elevator. When I return to the lab the others there are still storing the constantly appearing food in the freezer. There seem to be some very large roasts (possibly each a whole hind quarter's worth) being created now. As we continue to store the free meat for distribution to others I wake up.

118

Inner Work

06/30/98 – In A Futuristic Terminal (dream)

In a futuristic terminal waiting for a young passenger from the past. He arrives ashen white from fear. The journey to the future was swift and tumultuous for him. I pull him aside and listen as he describes a person he is looking for, a man with a leather coat with a large silver buckle. No one of that description gets off the shuttle. Finally, a young woman comes by wearing the jacket we ask her where she got it and she points to a man in the shadows. There is a sense of danger in the air as if several of the beings around us were assassins. We get into a transport that seems to be stopped at an intersection forever. As the danger looms nearer we finally stat to move. The car is like a roller coaster ride on tracks and moves swiftly over great arches and curves. One checks their seat belt for fear of falling out. At the end of the ride we get out and several beings make attempts to lunge at the child I am escorting. I am his protector as we journey onward to a foyer full of beings in conversation. The child notes how old everyone is and I remind him that he is older than all of us since he is in the future. We enter together into a large cavernous hall. It is a beautiful room with curved crystalline walls. A couple is in the center of the room giving birth to a male child named Jeremiah. They hand me a small bible with the child's name on the spine. Everyone in the hall seems to have a small bible in their hands each bearing a different name. Each bible contains a full life story past present and future of the name on the spine. The bible seems to only be able to be opened to the current instant in time, though you know that you can turn to any point in time after you have opened it. The bible each of us carry is for us to care for as we hold in our hands that soul's life. I sit in a chair against the wall and look in awe at the beauty of the cave. I set down the bible in my hand as I walk through a gallery of smaller caves to my left. Each small room is more beautiful than the one I leave, smooth crystal walls with soft warm colors washing over them from an unknown source, The colors seem to wave gently in time with the beautiful music emanating from around me. Each room has alcoves with smooth crystal figurines in them. Each more beautiful than the one before. A monk comes up to me and hands me the bible of Jeremiah I left behind. He places it softly in my hands as he warmly touches my hands. He says nothing though I sense he is telling me to keep the bible with me at all times and to enjoy the beauty of the caves. I keep wandering from room to room drinking in the beauty and love that emanates from the very depths of the crystalline walls. The figurines seem to be of Mary, Joseph, Jesus and all of the saints past present and future. There soft beauty soothes me as I wake up.

Inner Work

07/05/98 – In A Large Field Singing (dream)

In a large field, beautiful green rolling hills around, it is like a large picnic with many people. We are all singing and dancing, no musical instruments just people. If there needs to be music, we provide it by humming the sounds of the instrument required. The music is lively and happy. We are all dancing and enjoying the beautiful day. Everyone is very happy and full of love for one another. Smiles, hugs and kisses abound. Our souls seem to sing to each other.

07/23/98 – A Visit with Angels (dream)

With a group of people talking, someone says there is a fire at a home nearby. We go as we see the large flames in the distance. We thought the house was consumed as we neared the scene. I said no it is just a large tree in the yard on fire. As I spoke the fire jumped from the house to the tree. The house is unharmed, and the tree is engulfed in beautiful flames reaching the sky, but it is not damaged. Flames disappear as the scene changes. I am outside of a building that I need to enter. I am with a beautiful angelic seeming woman who can help me get in the building. She is my mother who passed away several years ago I tell the guard at the door. He enters with me, but others question how we got in. The guard introduces the woman to the people (they seem to be Xerox employees I know). He introduces the woman as Diana Mosten who died over a year ago. We go to an elevator and ride to the third floor. I notice that all the time I have been totally naked, but no one notices my nakedness in the presence of the angelic women. We get to the cafeteria where an employee is trying to put food away into a locked freezer. She cannot unlock the door and is worried the food will spoil. As I walk near, the door unlocks, and she opens it and thanks me for helping her. Three of us get into a small service elevator to go back down. I am explaining to the person with the woman and I about my visit with mom and Diana in Heaven. He looks bewildered, but I ask him if he has ever "seen" God. I tell him that I have been in God's presence with mom and Diana and that God's beauty can be only felt not really seen through our eyes. His beauty is brighter than the flames seen earlier that did not consume the house or the tree. There is a great sense of peace in the elevator as the wall opposite me bends toward me, so I can tap it to prove to the man with me that God is with us and that our world around us can be changed if only we try to make the changes. As the wall returns to its normal shape the door opens and we leave. It is just the guard and I in a beautiful field. A beautiful sunset is at our backs as a glorious rainbow arches across the sky before us. We are filled with a great sense of love and peace. I wake up felling God's love.

120

Inner Work

10/10/98 – A Transformation Occurs (dream)

Crouched near a curved wall hiding from people or beings that are searching for my friend and me. He is on the other side of the wall hiding near some trash cans. A couple of the beings come near as I tell my friend to hide with a wave of my hand. A trash collector comes by and sees me and my friend. He has his co-worker take the full can and he places a clean empty can next to my friend who gets in it. The collector takes the can across the street to a small doorway in a building. I stealthily follow. Outside the door I hear a commotion within and open the door. The creature who saved my friend was lying dead near the empty can. In a corner I see a green lizard or dragon that scurries through a hole in the wall to escape. The dragon's eyes look into mine and I notice he is my friend who has been transformed into this reptilian creature. He then disappears through the hole which seems to have been burnt through the wall by acidic saliva he spit on it. I leave the building feeling out of place with everything around me. I walk near a small hill and notice an old man dressed in a wizard's robe at the top of the hill. He seems to spin and dance, his feet barely touching the ground. As he twirls golden glitter or sparks seem to emanate from him in a swirl of color. He beckons to me and I begin to dance the same dance. Skipping and twirling in an Irish jig like dance down the street, In the middle of the square I jump up and notice that as I jump, I can float higher and higher with each jump. I can glide through the air at will. I float around the wizard's head and return to the ground. We go into a beautiful building on the top of the hill. We meet a man and woman who seem to be performers also. They are preparing to sing to the wizard's music as I dance. The man says he must enjoy his singing today as his voice is going. The woman looks sad as she confirms his truth. The wizard picks up a homemade instrument containing three wires strung on a wooden frame. He plucks the strings and beautiful music comes forth. The man and woman start to sing a beautiful lore ballad as I slowly dance on the balcony looking out over the peaceful valley below. I comment to the others that if I were ever to know I was ready to die or leave the world I was in that I would want to spend my last days here in this hideaway of peace and love surrounded by God's beauty. It is so wonderful here I keep saying as I glide around dancing, listening to the music. I wake up peaceful and full of love.

Inner Work

10/27/98 – A Need Is Felt (dream)

Standing in line ready to board an airplane, Sandy Patton, my dream partner, comes by and requests that I get out of line for a moment. She seems to be asking me to wait while she contacts Bob Stoudt to discuss her dreams. We sit down at a counter to talk. Sandy and I have been discussing our dreamwork ever since the last dream retreat we attended together. She has suggested that we take some time to work on dream analysis. I ask her how her pet skunk is, and she laughs. We should start the joint dreamwork soon I say. I feel that Sandy and I could start a small group of dream workers after discussing our own dreamwork. I wake up feeling that I need to contact Sandy to see what is going on in her dreamwork lately.

11/30/1998 –A Sensing Array (dream)

Reporting to a business in a tall office building, very futuristic in design. Company has an electronics lab that I am being given a tour of. Lead person is demonstrating a new piece of equipment that seems to be a large sensing array of some kind. As I observe there seems to be some kind of a problem getting the equipment started. I look over the array of electronic circuitry and touch a card that I feel is not functioning. They retry the demonstration and the equipment begins to function properly. The have video connection with several potential customers whom they have sent small scanner receiver/transmitter modules to for the test. As the equipment begins to cycle through its test sequence each customer site in order is observed. A visible wave passes through the corridor of the floor on which the sensor was placed, and data is sent back to the lab and a new wave is transmitted to the remote sensors. A resulting harmonious wave and comforting tone emanates from the remote unit and people in the rooms off the corridor are healed. I realize now that the customers sites are all critical care units in hospitals.

I am being given a tour of the lab by the director and he shows me into a large room full of very sophisticated computer driven electronic equipment. I am given a manual to review and as I touch the manual the symbols Alpha and Omega appear in my mind's eye and on the cover of the manual. The letters do not seem to be typed or printed on the manual only they seem to glow from within as I hold the book. I open the manual and read the detailed journal of the lab experiments and I then realize that the equipment was designed to sense electromagnetic imbalances in people caused by disease and emotional stress. The book speaks to electromagnetic and sound wave generation to effect healing in all living things within the range of the

122

scanner receiver/transmitters. The words speak of God's love for all of Mother/Father God's creation and how the new technology is being given to humankind to help heal the world. I have been chosen by the lab director to be part of the experiment because of my known development on the spiritual level. The test of my ability to assist in the work at hand was my touching the first equipment I was shown, and the equipment began to function. The director explained that only a few people had the proper inner peace and harmonious vibration to effect energizing of the delicate sensing equipment. He did not have to explain any further as I immediately became fully knowledgeable of the equipment's design and the task at hand.

The others began to take me on a complete tour of the facility. We walked into corridors that had smoky glass-like walls that were translucent, so one could see all around themselves. There seemed to be a beautifully landscaped park area in the court around which the building was built. The walls surrounding the courtyard were curved and smooth. The beauty of the park area was indescribable. It reminded me of the center of the Isle of Love and Life from my Journey Inward dream. As we walked through the pristine corridors, it seemed that we had to proceed through several doors in a proper sequence and speed or the passageways would become inaccessible. In several areas there were small alcoves facing the courtyard which contained equipment that sensed the area and sent data back to the main electronics. Everything seemed so delicately tuned and balanced that any anomaly would cause a reaction from the system. It was as if the equipment and God's creation were intricately linked in a symbiotic balance. As we approached one of the alcoves a tone began to emanate from the walls around us and my guide said we must hurry to open the door. As I reached for the door it seemed to respond to the presence of my hand before I reached it and opened to let us into the observation area. I stood there in the alcove staring in wonder at the beauty before me. I felt a wash of warmth and love pass over me as I woke up.

Inner Work

12/01/1998 – A Personal Observation

After rereading the last few months of my journal, I sat thinking of my life and the people around me; who they were and why they were given in presence to me by God.

I hope that this documentation of the last few years of dream work and analysis will help other men to face mid-life difficulties with a feeling of God's hand on their shoulder through the process. I fervently believe that God calls each and every one of us to look inward from time to time to review who we are and where we are heading.

The final two sections of this book are writings and observations of mine.

Poetry & Prose

06/06/76 –Jean, Jeanie

Jean, Jeanie ... Jean, Jeanie
Her name breathes through my heart
Like a soft spring breeze kissing life into the newborn leaves.
Her freshness is that of a thousand daffodils waving happily in a sun kissed field.
Her laughter fills my mind with memories.
Memories of all the beautiful things that have graced my past.

> The happy crinkle of the crust of a new fallen snow.
> The busy hum of bees working earnestly to create their sweet gift of honey.
> The soft whisper of a gentle breeze through tall pine majesty.
> The peaceful song of the first bird of spring announcing Mother Nature's splendor.
> The rustling of the multi-colored leaves on a brisk autumn morn.
> The overwhelming feeling of a love that must be told.
> Told to the stars, the world, the universe, and especially Jeanie.

Jean, Jeanie ... Jean, Jeanie
Her beauty rushes through my mind
Like a brisk summer rain awakening the sleeping flowers.
Her warmth is like a summer sun embracing the world and making all welcome.
Her eyes sparkle with life.

> Life enkindled within by a warm heart.
> A heart that I want for my own.
> Mine to cherish and love with devotion the rest of my life.
> Mine to share with nature's fair blessings.
> Blessings of health, happiness, and sunshine.
>> Health to help us enjoy our moments together.
>> Happiness to spread to all nearby.
>> And sunshine to brighten the path to the future.

Poetry and Prose

06/07/76 –Jean

I sleep without sleeping, I dream dreams of love. The image of Jean
swiftly passes my mind's eye. I await God's decision. Will I be blessed
or not? Will God allow my love to flourish or wither in the long days of
loneliness ">tween now and my next date with Jean.
Jean,
Jean,
Her name rings of beauty and love. In her is my future and my
dreams. Without her I am lost and wandering like an orphan in the
rain asking all who come near to understand but no one but Jean can.
Jean,
Jean,
Mother of Renee and Lee Ann, children of tomorrow.
Will they accept me as a protector?
Will they need me in times of fear?
Will they love me like true daughters?
Will they bring happiness to my years?
Only with Jean's help will this occur, with the gift of her help, I implore
God to bless me.
Jean,
Jean,
I love you!

06/08/76 –Wondering

Here I stand wondering, looking over the world from my balcony's perspective. Wondering, ever wondering, is life here so beautiful when the one you love is not here beside you. Can these sleepless nights be telling me something I should already know? Go Frank to your true love and win her heart for eternity." This deep feeling of loneliness for the arms that held me for those few short days, for the sweet lips that kissed mine and swiftly sent my heart on a merry chase for a lifetime of sharing. The picture of her face lingers on in my mind's eye, beautiful in every detail, copied to perfection in her daughters' youthful smiles. Happy will I be on the day I win her for my own. To compete for one's love is difficult, but it is a task I will endure until that time when I once again hold sweet Jean in my arms. This time never to let go until she is mine alone. Then there's Renee and Lee Ann, their mother's love radiates from them like soft summer breezes in the night air awakening the little boy in all men who come near to remember the joys of being so young and dependent. No worries, no cares for mother is always there but I for one wish to be there also as a proud parent watching his little girls grow up slowly, fighting the imaginary demons of the world in their sleep and crying out for two pairs of arms to protect them with their shelter of love. To hold mother and daughters in my arms during a soft evening rain and explain to them that the rain is a magic carpet of life awakening Mother Nature's plants so that all may enjoy her splendor. Especially Jean, Renee, Lee Ann and hopefully Frank.

06/10/76 –A Dream Come True

It was '76 the month was May
When I fell in love that day
I met a girl I'd often seen
But only in my fondest dreams
A gift from God my mind did say
But for her love I'd have to pray
A solemn vow I make this night
For this girl's love I'll always fight
And with the help of God above
I know I'll win my Jeanie's love.

Poetry and Prose

03/04/94 – I sit alone and in pain

I sit alone and in pain
My heart aches for Jean's love
I am changing daily
Becoming new, more aware
I am burying the old me
Death to controlling, overbearing Frank
I am seeking new inner life
Welcome to my soulmate, my anima
I pray for God's help
Open the inner doors to understanding
I ask for Jean's reconsideration
Reconsider the death of our bond
I want to explore last year
What really caused the rift
I hope Jack has a heart
Can he let Jean grow alone?
I love our family
They are being hurt deeply
I hope Jean's vision will clear
She does not see the family pain
I need Jean in my life
No one else could fill her space
I want an end to the waiting
We as a family need to talk
I am important to God
God blessed me with Jean
I can no longer bear the pain
Loneliness is crushing my soul
I am in conflict with myself
My anima is upset with me

Poetry and Prose

A vision of the Garden of Eden
(as described to me by Seth third son of Adam and Eve in a dream)

If you cross the misty mountains
then sail the azure sea
On the golden sand of love and hope
at the edge of time you'll see
The little girl named Phaedra
playing happily and free
If you softly ask her where you are
she'll show you 'round with glee
To the center of this isle of life
to a dale of emerald green
Where a majestic rainbow arching high
forever can be sees
'Neath the highest reaches of its bow
a grassy knoll so clean
Smothered in a veil of lilacs
the fragrance entices dreams
A pillar of pure alabaster
holds a book as old as time
There words inscribed by God's own hand
bring visions to your mind
The pages talk of love and life
with a mate so gentle and kind
Enraptured by the story
you leave stress and strife behind
The images so vivid
fill your soul with inner peace
One cannot help but wonder
who prepared this soulful feast
Phaedra waves her arms in a heart shaped move
and points you toward the East
There inscribed in ivory by pen of gold
are poems from the past
As the book of love and life is held
firmly in your grasp
The image of a perfect mate
'cross your mind's eye softly slips
There stands a bride in radiant white
love's smile upon her lips
You take her hand as Phaedra
guides you to your wedding ship

Upon which you'll journey ever more
God's love will guide your trip
Your bond of love is written
in the pages of that book
God's hand has blessed each marriage
His kingdom can't be shook
To reaffirm those marriage vows
one must chance to take a look
Into each other's heart to find
love's scripture in that book.

Poetry and Prose

03/29/94 –The Dark Side of the Isle

A vision of the Sin of Man
(as described to me by Seth third son of Adam and Eve in a dream)

A dark side exists to the Isle of Love and Life
Where the evil mother brews a mixture of strife
Where loneliness and pain constantly dance
Sad comment on love's sacred stance
Here demons play, and chaos starts
Crushing love and life from foolish hearts
Phaedra warns of dangers on that side
But loves blind rush enjoys the ride
On chariots of doom into the dreary night
To save our souls we must ever fight
The tempting urge of the demon's song
And return to center where we belong
The dark side's lure is reckless fun
We close our hearts to everyone
Except those who ride the chariot of doom
For timeless love there is no room
We forsake the love of family and friend
As temptations larger than life amend
Our thoughts and dreams of others fond
And make sacrifice of love's true bond
The vortex pulls us into the pit
A dark dank hole in which we sit
Pray God to help us find the light
To guide us back on a path that's right
Phaedra awaits to lead us home
We only need to reach for the tome
The book of love and life it seems
Can return us to our pleasant dreams
We must take time to stop and look
At love's sacred verse in God's own book
To inward look and softly pray
For God's blessed guidance on the way
To journey out from stress and strain
To play on the golden sand again

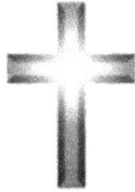

06/22/94 – Musings on Death
by Frank J. Costanza

Is death the end of life or the beginning of eternity?
If it is an end of life then why strive for unattainable goals,
Why chance romance, love or relationship during your short passage through.
Death is the beginning of the more complete love relationship with God.
It opens the door to your soul's fulfillment of its ultimate purpose:
To bring you into total communion with God, to allow you to taste the fruits of your full and rich life. Death in itself seems painful to those left behind mainly because their souls also long to reach that final plateau of love and connection with God. The souls of those left behind share their pain with each other because they know where the departed person's soul has gone. We as people do not comprehend that level of existence where time is put aside, and eternity begins and ends, was and is; a timeless expanse of infinite dimensions where souls can connect and learn all there is to learn, feel all there is to feel, love all there is to love and be one with God in divine light.

Poetry and Prose

11/06/94 – All Saints Sunday Sermon

Good morning let each of us ponder for a moment what today is, All Saints Sunday. Let's try to picture in our minds eye the saints. Close your eyes for a moment, picture in your mind's eye what the saints look like. Now that you've had time to think, what was the image that you saw? Did most of us see someone in a long flowing white robe with a halo above their head? Or, did someone see their parents, their neighbor, or someone sitting near them and say to themselves Saint Anne, Saint Chris, etc. Or, did you see yourselves as saints. I think of the saints and I think of my parents because these are people who, no matter what we did as children, right or wrong, they still loved us, just as God loves us as His children no matter what we do, right or wrong. We are all saints in God's eyes. From that moment of conception, creation starts one more time and another beginning starts on the face of this earth, God has made that entity a saint. God doesn't say, "To be a saint one must belong to this church or that church." God loves all of His creation and as such we are all saints. As Martin Luther taught us we are both saint and sinner. We are all forgiven all of our sins because we are God's children. In today's readings we listen to the Beatitudes. Many people have trouble with the way the beatitudes are written. Picture yourself as an apostle or a Pharisee, one of those who have done everything right, paid their tithe, followed Jesus, gave to the poor, fed the hungry, did everything possible that they could to be good and do right and then they hear Jesus Christ say to them:

"Blessed are the poor in spirit, for theirs is the kingdom of heaven."
"Blessed are those who mourn, for they will be comforted."
"Blessed are the meek, for they will inherit the earth."
"Blessed are those who hunger and thirst for righteousness, for they will be filled."
"Blessed are the merciful, for they will receive mercy."
"Blessed are the pure in heart, for they will see God."
"Blessed are the peacemakers, for they will be called children of God."
"Blessed are those who are persecuted for righteousness' sake, for theirs is the kingdom of heaven."
"Blessed are you when people revile you and persecute you and utter all kinds of evil against you falsely on my account. Rejoice and be glad, for your reward is great in Heaven, for in the same way they persecuted the prophets who were before you."

Does this mean that one must be poor in spirit, in mourning, meek, full of pain and suffering, always merciful and always pure in heart, peacemakers, persecuted and reviled at all times to be able to see God? I think not, I think what Christ was telling the apostles was that everyone is Blessed in His Father's eyes, even those who are following Him through the mountains and deserts who are saying "Lord I am not

134

worthy!" He is saying to them "Yes you are, you are children of God, you are all worthy."

"Blessed are the peacemakers." Who are the peacemakers? Are they the people in Washington, D.C. and the other capitols of the world who make laws and write peace treaties? No, not just them but everyone who shows love for one another and themselves. Let me give you an example of peacemakers in my life. I was raised by two beautiful people, my parents, and many a time, "MANY A TIME", my brothers and I or my sisters and I got into arguments or fights and yelled all kinds of things at each other and mom and dad were there as peacemakers. They were there for us. Many times, the older child is the peacemaker amongst the younger children of the family and vice versa. We are all peacemakers, sometime in our lives. We are all saints even though we are also sinners.

We all join around this communion table on Sundays to share God's gifts and on this Sunday, "All Saints Sunday", we take special time to remember those who have been, and are, most important in our lives, living or dead. Pastor Reeves once told me she enjoys Eucharist so much because this is the time that she can be around the table once again with her late husband and share Sunday dinner with him. I think that's beautiful. I would like to expand on that thought for each of us in light of the Beatitudes. We have all mourned in our lives at one time or other for the loss of a loved one or friend through death, be it by sickness, old age or even suicide. Two years ago, at this time my family was preparing for a great celebration, the fiftieth anniversary of my mom and dad's marriage. On November 28, 1992 we had a grand party, mom and dad renewed their wedding vows, I was dad's best man as his had passed away. I stood there on the altar and witnessed their great love for one another. We all went to their reception and partied hearty in celebration of the long life together. Mom and dad danced like Fred and Ginger. A week later, on December 5th, my mom had a heart attack and died the next day, three days before my birthday. I was angry at her for leaving me just before my birthday. I was angry at God for taking her away, but it was her time to go. I was the one who talked to the family priest and let him know she had passed away. He gave me the option to choose the day of her burial and I chose my birthday, so that, on my forty-seventh birthday, I was able to say goodbye to mom one final time in a place she loved most, her church. Other people in my life have passed on also, my favorite uncle died several months later, and his family was hurt and angry that he should be taken away from them. As a Marine I had a best friend who committed suicide in boot camp because he could not qualify on the rifle range. Kind of a dumb reason for killing oneself. His death hurt me deeply and I was angry. In Viet Nam another friend committed suicide and I was mad at him, maybe because he found a way out of there, but not the way I wanted and not the way I did. In Viet Nam I lost many friends and saw more death than I ever wished to see in my life. God has always helped me through these losses by giving me the ability to understand that death is not the end. It is the beginning of a more complete love relationship with God, no matter how one dies. It opens the door to the departed soul's fulfillment of its ultimate purpose. It brings the soul into total communion with God to allow the departed to taste the fruits of their full rich life, however long that life existed on earth. Those of us left behind feel the hurt and pain of loss and we must make peace with that pain and realize that we are still very much connected with those departed souls and that they are with us at all times. They have gone to a new level of existence where time is put aside, and eternity begins and ends, was and is; a timeless expanse of infinite dimensions where souls connect and learn all there is to learn, feel all there is to feel, love all there is to love and become one with God in His divine light. We must go beyond our hurt and anger when we lose someone we care about in our life, not only through death but through divorce or separation, or through a stupid argument with a friend that turns him or her cold to us for months or maybe even years. We must make peace with that hurt and go on. All losses are very painful and hurt and we mourn, so we all mourn, sometime in our life. We are all peacemakers, sometime in our life. We are all poor in spirit, sometime in our life. We are all meek, sometime in our life. Maybe we should all remember those people who have departed or those people who are not in our lives any more when we come to communion and take that pain that is inside us, that anger and hurt, and place it on this table and offer it up to God. I would love to have my mother here with me, Uncle Leo, my Marine friends, many who died in Viet Nam. I would love to have them all around this table with me, and I do because, as it says in the apostle's creed "I believe in the communion of saints" and as we gather around this table remember, we are sharing Sunday dinner with all the saints in heaven and on earth. AMEN

Poetry and Prose

03/15/95 –"THANK YOU, GOD, I LOVE YOU!"

Good morning, my name is Frank Costanza, I have been a member here at Saint Timothy's for about six years and I am honored to be given the privilege to speak to you today about stewardship. I would like to tell you about how I was taught about stewardship as a child. My father was Lutheran, and my mother was Roman Catholic, as such my brothers, sisters and I were raised in the Catholic Church. Our parents taught us to give to the church by their example coupled with the church's help. I remember as a child at Catechism class, our Sunday School held on Saturday mornings, receiving our weekly offering envelopes for collection at church on Sunday. Back then my allowance was ten cents a week which I promptly went out to the local five and dime and bought a bag of candy (wax teeth and lips, some bubble gum, a couple of licorice whips, etc.). For nine cents you could get a bag of candy to last several days if rationed properly and the penny change went into the envelope for church (10% of my allowance.) Some weeks when times were difficult, we received no allowance, so my envelope was empty. I felt it important to give something to God on Sunday so when I had no money, I wrote a note saying, "Thank you God, I love you." and put it in my envelope for collection. As a child I had learned to tithe but, as I grew older and earned more and became responsible for my own expenses, I also began to rationalize the value of my time as part of my giving to the church and the monetary amount became less and less of my real income. I also started to control my giving depending on my attitude towards my pastor, church council, or others at church. I had lost sight of the real reason for giving to God. Tithing is for God's work and human differences or difficulties should be set aside when preparing one's gift to God. How easy it is to find enough spare cash to buy a six pack of beer to watch a ball game with, to pay green fees for another eighteen holes of golf, to get your hair done one extra time, to rent a couple of movies or video games, or to pay for any other of a multitude of selfish wants and needs when one doesn't pay God his due first. I lost sight of what my father always taught me, "Don't ever let your personal life come between you and God, remember people are human and God is God. First give your gift to God and God will provide." My father sits down weekly to do his bills usually on Saturday mornings, allowance day when I was growing up. I used to sit and watch him sometimes. He would write in his deposit from Friday's paycheck, balance his checkbook then write out his check for church for 10% or more of his deposit, place it in his Sunday offering envelope then proceed to pay what bills he could pay with the rest. I only wish I had learned his discipline. While contemplating this talk I thought of my childhood, my family, and this church family so full of love and came up with a way to help myself to give better to God and maybe this idea would be useful to all of us. As you open your checkbook to write your check out for the offertory, before writing anything else on the check, in the memo space at the bottom write "Thank you God or I love you God." say a short prayer of thanks sign your name then write in the amount from your heart. If each of us were to give up just one of our little gifts to ourselves each week and offered it up to God, together we would be able to fight this deficit our church faces. Remember God loves all of us no matter who we are or what we do so can't we each give a little more to help God's church.

"THANK YOU, GOD, I LOVE YOU!"

04/17/95 – Doubting Thomas Sermon

Good Morning today is low Sunday, in the gospel today we listen to the story of Thomas, the twin. He is known to us as Doubting Thomas because here is a man who spent years walking with Christ, learning from Christ, watching the miracles of Christ and when he is told by his friends that Christ returned and talked to them after He arose from the dead he said, "No way, I don't believe *that*; show me. Let me see the wounds in His hands. Let me see the wound in His side. Let me touch them; let me put my fingers and hand in them. Then I will believe. " Just think; the amount of doubt that that man had, even though he was with Christ all along, and saw what Christ could do, still he doubted. But didn't they all doubt? Didn't the apostles push aside the witness given by the women who talked with the angels at the tomb as idle chatter? Didn't they ALL doubt?

Now let's consider the life of Christ Thomas was witness to and ask ourselves, "Why did God pick 2,000 years ago for this to happen? What if He'd chosen now instead of 2,000 years ago? Can you imagine what the last six weeks would have been like with today's media coverage? There would be hidden cameras in the Garden, watching Christ as He did His praying and thinking and talking with the Apostles, waking them up. Can you imagine what these last TWO weeks would have been like? Can you imagine Oprah, Geraldo, Sally Jesse Raphael, Montel, all those TV talk show people? Oh, they would have the time of their lives. The shows they would bombard us with; "Jesus Christ, Son of God or Master of Illusion, " "The Abandoned Families of the Apostles, " "Mary and Joseph, The Inside Story, " "An Interview with Mary Magdalene, " the topics would be endless. The stories they would have; There would be a panel of illusionists such as David Copperfield and Siegfried discussing the secrets behind Christ's miracles. "Water into wine, appearing in a locked room, mere parlor tricks, I walked through the Great Wall of China. " David Copperfield would say. They would attack the reasoning of the apostles. They would troop one after another of the apostle's families on TV saying, "Oh, those terrible men! Look what they have done. They left their families -- cast them aside to follow this other person through the desert. To listen to Him, to watch Him pray, to learn from Him. And leave their families stranded? To leave them alone to survive on their own? Without the breadwinner here, without anyone to bring food to the family. How could they treat their own flesh and blood like that? "

Ah yes, the apostles would have been taken over the coals. And what about this man Jesus Christ? Would the press have fun with the camera coverage of His trial. The last two weeks would have been a production -- a Cecil B. DeMille type production -- O. J. Simpson's trial would be nothing compared to what they would do with TV coverage of this man's trial. Christ's trial certainly would not last only one day. The jury selection alone would take months. There would be so many secrets brought out in the open. Everybody would know who did what, who was where. Do you think Peter would be able to deny his presence? There would be camera reviews of where Christ was at all different times – "Yes, there he is! Him, Peter, the man talking with the one called Jesus Christ. Photographic and video tape evidence. People seeing him there right on camera. Peter could not deny Christ.

Do you believe for one moment that in today's judicial system Christ could be convicted and put to death? I think not. The lawyers would fight over the opportunity to defend this man in court. If convicted the appeal process and stays of execution would prolong the inevitable. Would WE allow ourselves to be cleansed of sin and saved by crying out "Let Him be crucified! "? Or would we stand by the sidelines and watch the drama unfold in the comfort of our homes and be at best disinterested third parties?

Ah, yes. It would have been a different story if Christ had been born in this time rather than 2,000 years ago. It would have been a very different story. I would have to believe that IF Christ had been found guilty and crucified that the day of His Resurrection would have been a Stephen Spielberg presentation, the best and most glorious presentation you could ever imagine. A production beyond all belief. The broadcast teams would have cameras focused on His tomb from every conceivable angle. We would have sat at home or in our local pub and watched it all on national TV, with our full six-foot-wide screens, watching, waiting for the great Resurrection of Christ, our savior.

Just think. What would it have been like if God chose OUR time to bring His Son down to Earth? I think it would have been amazing, but would it have been the same? If it were the United States, you know Thomas and the other apostles would have come from Missouri, the "Show Me" state!

And how about us? How about you and me? How would we take this man Jesus Christ walking around, selecting a few leaders to follow Him and say, "You are my apostles; we are going to build a whole new Church, a whole new spiritual way of life? "? Would this man not be just torn apart on TV? What would the press say? The Star, The Inquirer ... boy, we would know all the secrets real or fabricated.

140

Think about why God chose 2,000 years ago instead of today. Because today the story of Thomas doubting would not be the same. The ability of the apostles to walk away from their families and trust that their families would be taken care of by friends and neighbors would not be the same.

Those men followed Christ to form a whole new way of living. And yes, Thomas doubted, as did all the apostles but he did not have the advantages of today's media events. The apostles could have tape recorded Christ's return to them in their locked room. The women at the tomb could have recorded the angel's message. But they could not do that 2,000 years ago. Back then you had to believe, you had to have undying faith.

Today, even with all the media coverage you could possibly have, even watching everything as it happened, with people on the scene as witnesses, we would still have our doubting Thomases. We would still have OUR doubts. Would we be able to be like the other apostles, or would the majority of us be like Thomas? Would it have to be proven by Christ standing in front of us? Would we say, "Show me??? "
What do you think your choice would be? AMEN

Poetry and Prose

04/02/96 – An Apology to God
Frank James Costanza

I write my apologies on the wind
　　To the one above who never sinned
He leads me on with fire within
　　To preach His word and share again
The inner work we each must do
　　To find the drive to start anew
Looking inward for forces true
　　To accomplish all God asks us to
To change the lives and ways of all
　　To answer God's unwavering call
To spread the word and prove appall
　　At mankind's invention of a fall
Since time began on this fair earth
　　Humankind has questioned its own true worth
I profess we must discard this dearth
　　Life with God within is one of mirth
A life so whole and full of grace
　　That one can bear the darkest place
The worst life offers we can face
　　When God's love within sets the pace
Forgiveness is a virtue found
　　Love and care shall then abound
God's grace always will astound
　　As ever onward we will bound
Moving toward that final day
　　When all will come to see God's way
To join together and prayerfully say
　　With God in heaven we are one today

Poetry and Prose

05/11/97 – LOVE

The Etymology of Mother
Written in honor of Mary Elizabeth Carvey Costanza
by Frank James Michael Costanza
May 11, 1997

Love, its labor creates a child that lights a mother's life
 A child so small and fragile snuggling at her breast
  As a mother holds and cuddles her child she feels so good inside
  A smile of thanks to God appears when baby says, "MA MA"

Observing a child grow brings warmth to a mother's smile
 First words, first steps, other memories fill the mother's heart
  The child grows more each day with mother there to guide
  The stages change, and "MA MA" now becomes "MOMMY"

Volumes have been written about the teenage year's turmoil
 But mother's love sustains and helps the child to grow
  The fears a mother feels as her child grows more aware
  Are somewhat pushed behind when "MOMMY" turns to "MOM!"

Even the great women of our times struggle with their children's growth
 They watch and hope and pray as the child becomes adult
  They feel the loss of need as their child goes to the world
  Alone with great strength inside and "MOM!" is now "MOTHER"

Personal Contact with GOD

Spring of 1958 – A Vision of Michael the Archangel

Part of the process of preparing for confirmation in the Roman Catholic Church is the selection of one's confirmation name. All of my friends had selected their confirmation names and I was the only one who had not made a choice. The selection had to be a name that meant something to each of us and we had to explain to our confirmation teacher why we chose who we did. Time was running out on me as I still found no name to choose. A particularly restful night, as I recall, was interrupted by a voice calling to me at the foot of my bed. I half awoke and saw a vision of a male figure standing there encircled in a brilliant glow. As he spoke, I noticed wings upon his back. He said to me, "I am Michael the Archangel, God assigned me when you were born to be your guardian angel. I am here now because you are troubled with your choice of a name. Use mine if you wish. " I knew at that moment that Michael was to be my confirmation name. I told my teacher of my selection the next Saturday during class and explained my vision. He did not altogether believe what I said happened, but I believed and that was what counted to me. I was confirmed Frank James Michael Costanza in Quantico, Virginia by the military prelate Francis Cardinal Spellman.

Personal Contact with God

Summer 1975 – Aunt Minnie's Farm, Stumptown, WV

The end of a long and fun-filled Bluegrass Festival weekend and we start our journey home. It is 2 AM on Monday when we decide to stop for a short rest on a beautiful overlook in the Shenandoah Valley region. There is no moon, no man-made lights to be seen, nothing but a clear star-filled sky, soft gentle breezes wafting through the trees and a feeling that all is right with the world. Millard and I stop our car and sit on a picnic table in the clearing and open a couple of beers and start to play music and sing. This is my first attempt at playing the harmonica and I enjoy playing along with Millard's guitar. As we play several people stop on their way home from the festival and bring out their instruments and join us. By 3:30 there are at least 24 of us playing familiar songs and singing in the beautiful night air. We start making up a song praising God. We make up a chorus then take turns creating verses. After about the third versa something beautiful begins to happen as each person begins to sing their new verse. No sooner does the first word of their personal verse of praise begin then all of us sing the complete verse as if we had the words written down in front of us. This goes on until the break of dawn when we decide to stop singing and hit the road home. We all feel as though God had touched us deeply and there is a camaraderie between us that is unexplainable. A group of 24 people from various different states and walks of life had just shared several hours of praise to God and became very connected to each other. I believe that there was a definite presence of God on that mountainside that morning and I will never forget the feeling of absolute peace and friendship we all felt the beautiful Summer of 1975.

Personal Contact with God

June First, 1984 – God cures Anthony

Anthony Charles Costanza was born at 1:01 PM May 30, 1984. It was to be a joyous family occasion. Jean and I had been through the required Lamaze classes for natural childbirth and Renee, Lee Ann and Michael had been prepared for attending Anthony's birth in the family birthing room at Rhinebeck Hospital. The birth was going along perfectly except for Jean's back labor and we were all excited to see the top of Anthony's head appear. As he was being delivered, he twisted several times and the umbilical cord became wrapped around his neck three times. As he was delivered, he looked like a limp doll and the nurse immediately rushed him into the next room and started giving him oxygen. They respirated him for 27 minutes before he finally breathed on his own and he appeared out of the woods. The next morning at 5:55 AM I was called to come to the hospital as he was going to be transported to Albany Medical Center due to seizure activity during the night. I called Father Frank Malau to meet me at the hospital to see Tony. I had Frank baptize Tony in his incubator just to be safe. At Albany Medical Center we are told the he may be there for several weeks until the seizure activity subsided. I left for home very upset at the prospect of my son being mentally handicapped for life. During Lent earlier I said morning prayer daily at church and continued it every day since for some reason. Friday morning, I stopped at church to say my morning prayers and ask God's help with Anthony. Above the altar at Saint James Episcopal Church in Hyde Park, New York is a beautiful circular stained-glass window with the dove of peace signifying the Holy Spirit in it. As the sun breaks through the window at 6:35 AM and shines upon my pained face I feel two hands on my shoulders (I am alone in the church) and hear God's voice say, "Go in peace your child is healthy." I feel greatly relieved and rush to Albany to see Tony. I relate my experience to his doctors who seem skeptical about my experience except for Dr. Pete who believes me because as we look on Anthony's medical chart, we notice that the last recorded seizure was at 6:34 AM. God had indeed interceded and blessed us with a healthy child.

www.ingramcontent.com/pod-product-compliance
Lightning Source LLC
Chambersburg PA
CBHW070935030426
42336CB00014BA/2679